Praise for OVERCOMING BINGE EATING

"By any standard, Dr. Fairburn is the leading authority in our field, so who better to write the definitive book on binge eating? This program is based on vast clinical experience, numerous clinical trials, and a breadth of perspective that few possess. You can trust this book. It is a landmark."
>—*Kelly D. Brownell, PhD, coauthor of* Food Fight;
>*Director, Rudd Center for Food Policy and Obesity,*
>*Yale University*

"Readers have posted online calling the previous version of this book 'a godsend' and 'the best book out there.' This substantially revised second edition is as good as the first and sets the standard for self-help books. This clearly written, practical guide is invaluable for anyone suffering from binge eating problems."
>—*Roz Shafran, PhD, Professor of Clinical Psychology,*
>*University of Reading, United Kingdom*

"This invaluable second edition incorporates recent advances in the treatment of binge eating, including new strategies for dealing with body image issues. I recommend this user-friendly book wholeheartedly."
>—*G. Terence Wilson, PhD, Oscar K. Buros Professor*
>*of Psychology, Rutgers, The State University of New Jersey*

"It is hard to improve a classic, but that is exactly what Dr. Fairburn has done. *Overcoming Binge Eating, Second Edition,* expands on the author's highly effective treatment. This self-help guide is filled with specific tools that can help reverse unhealthy habits that have trapped you for years. Dr. Fairburn helps you maintain regular eating habits, distract yourself from cravings, stop emotional eating, and address body image issues. My colleagues and I will be recommending this book to all of our clients who feel their eating is out of control."
>—*Robert L. Leahy, PhD, author of* The Worry Cure

"In this gem of a book, now thoroughly revised, Dr. Fairburn draws on decades of clinical experience and research. This is a powerful resource for anyone who wants to achieve lasting self-change."
>—*Ruth H. Striegel, PhD, Editor-in-Chief,*
>International Journal of Eating Disorders

OVERCOMING BINGE EATING

Overcoming Binge Eating

SECOND EDITION

The Proven Program to Learn Why
You Binge and How You Can Stop

DR. CHRISTOPHER G. FAIRBURN

THE GUILFORD PRESS
New York   London

© 2013 The Guilford Press
A Division of Guilford Publications, Inc.
370 Seventh Avenue, Suite 1200, New York, NY 10001
www.guilford.com

Part II © 2013 Christopher G. Fairburn

Printed in the United States of America

This book is printed on acid-free paper.

Last digit is print number: 9   8   7   6   5   4   3

Library of Congress Cataloging-in-Publication Data

Fairburn, Christopher G.
      Overcoming binge eating : the proven program to learn why you binge
and how you can stop / Christopher G. Fairburn. — Second edition.
          pages   cm
      Includes bibliographical references and index.
      ISBN 978-1-57230-561-8 (pbk.) — ISBN 978-1-4625-1044-3 (hardcover)
      1. Compulsive eating—Popular works.   I. Title.
      RC552.C65F35 2013
      616.85'26—dc23
                                                                            2013011365

To Kristin, George, and Henry;
Guy, Sarah, and Susan

I want to acknowledge those who have helped
me most in my career:

Michael Gelder, Robert Kendell,
Zafra Cooper, and Terry Wilson

My past and present colleagues at the
Centre for Research on Eating Disorders
at Oxford (CREDO)

The Wellcome Trust

Acknowledgments

Overcoming Binge Eating is a book for people with binge eating problems, and it has been written with their help. I therefore want to start by thanking those patients and volunteers who commented on early versions of the book and tested out the self-help program. Their contributions were invaluable. In addition, I want to thank the friends and colleagues who helped me create the forerunner of the present book. I am particularly indebted to Kelly Brownell, Jacqui Carter, Zafra Cooper, Phillipa Hay, Laura Hill, Marsha Marcus, Marianne O'Connor, and Terry Wilson.

This new version of *Overcoming Binge Eating* was written with the input of Emma Clifton, Sarah Squire, and Suzanne Straebler. I am enormously grateful to all three of them. I am also grateful to Natalie Barnes, Mara Catling, and Sarah Collins for their careful proofreading.

Lastly, I want to thank the Wellcome Trust. This extraordinary foundation has funded me and my research since 1984. Without its support this self-help program, and the treatment upon which it is based, would never have been developed.

Contents

Purchasers may download and print select practical
tools from this book at *www.credo-oxford.com*.

Introduction

This Book and How to Use It

If you have a problem controlling your eating, this book is for you—whatever your age, whatever your gender, and whatever your weight. *Overcoming Binge Eating* will provide you with a readable and authoritative account of binge eating problems and how to overcome them. Part I presents the most current facts while Part II comprises a self-help program based on the latest version of the most effective treatment available. This "enhanced" program can be used by anyone with a binge eating problem so long as he or she is not substantially underweight (see p. 124).

The original version of *Overcoming Binge Eating* was published in 1995. Since then Part I has become established as a trustworthy source of information on binge eating problems. Meanwhile the treatment program in Part II has been investigated in numerous clinical trials, making it possibly the most extensively tested self-help program for any problem. Time after time it has been found to be a potent source of help, either when used on its own or when used with external support (guided self-help). As a result the program has become established as a leading treatment for binge eating problems. In recognition of this, *Overcoming Binge Eating* was awarded a Seal of Merit from the U.S. Association for Behavioral and Cognitive Therapies, and in the U.K. National Health Service doctors can prescribe the book as if it were a form of medication.

But time moves on, new knowledge is acquired, and with the new knowledge comes advances in treatment. As a result this version of *Overcoming Binge Eating* is essentially a new book. I have thoroughly revised Part I to ensure it continues to provide a comprehensive and up-to-date account of what we know about binge eating problems. It now addresses all types of binge eating problems including those seen in anorexia nervosa. It also provides much more information about dieting, body weight, and body image.

I have also substantially modified Part II in light of advances in treatment and in particular the development of a new "enhanced" version of the trustworthy evidence-based treatment. CBT-E includes a new way of conceptualizing eating problems, improved ways of regaining control over eating, a more sophisticated approach to the addressing of concerns about shape and weight, and much more emphasis on relapse prevention. These new developments have been incorporated into the self-help program. The program in this version of *Overcoming Binge Eating* is, in essence, a self-help version of CBT-E.

If you have a binge eating problem, you may be tempted to go straight to Part II of the book. This would be a mistake. You need to read Part I first (at a minimum read Chapters 1, 4, and 5) as this will help you understand your problem and why it has become so self-perpetuating. This understanding is essential if you are to benefit from the self-help program. On the other hand, you may be unsure whether you have a binge eating problem. If this is the case, I suggest you read the very same key chapters (Chapters 1, 4, and 5) in Part I to see if you identify with the problems described. If you do, then move on to the beginning of Part II (p. 119), where I discuss the pros and cons of attempting to change.

PART I

Binge Eating Problems
The Facts

CHAPTER 1

Binge Eating

It starts off with my thinking about the food that I deny myself when I am dieting. This soon changes into a strong desire to eat. First of all it is a relief and a comfort to eat, and I feel quite high. But then I can't stop, and I binge. I eat and eat frantically until I am absolutely full. Afterwards I feel so guilty and angry with myself.

This book has been written for anyone who has a problem controlling their eating, whatever their age, whatever their gender, whatever their weight. It is about eating in an uncontrolled way. It is about binge eating.

The term *binge* used to mean one thing to most people: drinking to excess. Today the word more often means eating to excess. For many people a binge is something perfectly innocuous—a dietary slip or lapse, a simple overindulgence. For others, though, it signifies partial or complete loss of control over eating. This is a major problem for a large number of people, and not just those in the Western world.

Yet despite the fact that binge eating is undeniably widespread, most people know comparatively little about the problem. Are binges always large? Are they always followed by purging? Is binge eating a lifelong problem, or can it be overcome? Is binge eating a sign that something else is wrong? What sort of person is prone to binge and why? How do we distinguish—in ourselves or in those we care about—between a true binge and simple overeating? And, most important of all, how can people learn to overcome binge eating?

None of these questions can be answered without a full under-standing of what a binge is, and that is the subject of this opening chapter.

WHAT DOES *BINGE* MEAN?

The meaning of the word *binge* has changed over the years. It has been in common use since the mid-nineteenth century when *binge* meant principally "a heavy drinking bout, hence a spree," accord-ing to the *Oxford English Dictionary*. While that remains one of its meanings, nowadays dictionaries often define a binge in terms of overeating, and the term *indulgence* may be used. *Merriam Webster's Collegiate Dictionary*, Eleventh Edition, for example, says that one meaning of the word *binge* is "an unrestrained and often excessive indulgence."

This so-called "indulgence" is actually a common phenom-enon reported by both men and women. For some it is an occasional indiscretion, as mentioned earlier; it has no effect on their lives. For others, though—such as the woman whose description opened this chapter—it is a genuine problem, something that has a profound impact on many aspects of their lives. Failure to understand this dis-tinction—between indulgence and binge eating—lies at the heart of much of the confusion about the behavior.

Recognizing the need to clarify the meaning of the term *binge eating*, researchers have investigated the experiences of those who binge eat. While no two personal accounts are identical, it turns out that the episodes of eating that people view as binges have two core features in common: The amount eaten is viewed as excessive—although it might not seem so to the outsider—and, crucially, there is a sense of loss of control at the time. It is important to be aware that technical definitions of a binge generally specify an additional feature, namely, that the amount eaten was definitely larger than most

> *Binges have two features in common: the amount eaten is viewed as excessive, and there is a sense of loss of control at the time.*

people would eat under similar circumstances. This size requirement is somewhat contentious, as we will discuss later in this chapter, but it is widely employed.

THE CHARACTERISTICS OF A BINGE

I randomly grab whatever food I can and push it into my mouth, sometimes not even chewing it. But I then start feeling guilty and frightened as my stomach begins to ache and my temperature rises. It is only when I feel really ill that I stop eating.

Personal descriptions of binge eating can be tremendously revealing. What emerges is an account that you might recognize if you binge or someone you know binges.

Feelings. The first moments of a binge can be pleasurable. The taste and texture of the food may seem intensely enjoyable. Such feelings seldom last long, however. Soon they are replaced by feelings of disgust as the person consumes more and more food. Some people feel revulsion over what they are doing but nevertheless continue to eat.

Speed of Eating. Typically people eat rapidly during a binge. Many people stuff food into their mouth almost mechanically, barely chewing it. Some also drink copiously to help wash the food down, which contributes to their feeling full and bloated. Drinking a lot also helps people bring up the food later on.

Agitation. Some people pace up and down or wander around during their binges. They may exhibit an air of desperation. They feel the craving for food as a powerful force that drives them to eat. This is why the term "compulsive eating" is sometimes used. Obtaining food may take on extreme importance; people may take food belonging to others, shoplift from stores, or eat discarded food. Most view such behavior as shameful, disgusting, and degrading.

I begin by having a bowl of cereal. I eat it really quickly and then immediately have two or three more bowls. By then I know that my control is blown and that I am going to go all the way and binge. I still feel very tense, and I desperately search for food. These days this means running around college looking for food people have thrown out. I know that this is really disgusting. I stuff the food down quickly. Sometimes I go into town, stopping at stores along the way. I buy only a little from each store so as not to arouse suspicion. I stop when I have run out of money or, more usually, because I am so full that I physically cannot eat any more.

A Feeling of Altered Consciousness. People often describe feeling as if they are in a trance during a binge. If you have experienced this trance-like state, you know that your behavior seems almost automatic, as if it is not really you who is eating. But, like the person below, people also report that they watch television, listen to loud music, or engage in some other form of distraction to prevent them from having to think about what they are doing.

It all starts with the way I feel when I wake up. If I am unhappy or someone has said something to upset me, I feel a strong urge to eat. When this urge comes, I feel hot and clammy. My mind goes blank, and I automatically move toward food. I eat really quickly, as if I'm afraid that by eating slowly I will have too much time to think about what I am doing. I eat standing up or walking around. I often eat watching television or reading a magazine. This is all to prevent me from thinking, because thinking would mean facing up to what I am doing.

Secretiveness. A hallmark of the typical binge is that it occurs in secret. Some people are so ashamed of their binge eating that they go to great lengths to hide it—and may succeed for many years. One way they accomplish this is by eating in a relatively normal manner when they are with others. Another is by exercising considerable subterfuge. Perhaps you are familiar with some of the ways that people keep their behavior hidden: for example, after eating a normal meal, some people later return surreptitiously to eat all the leftovers. Others take food to their bedroom or bathroom to eat it without fear of detection.

> *I leave work and go shopping for food. I begin eating before I get home, but it is in secret with the food hidden in my pockets. Once I'm home, proper eating begins. I eat until my stomach hurts and I cannot eat any more. It is only at this point that I snap out of my trance and think about what I have done.*

Loss of Control. As mentioned earlier, the experience of being out of control is one of the two core features of binge eating. It is what distinguishes binge eating from everyday overeating. The experience varies considerably between people. Some feel it long before they begin eating. For others it emerges gradually as they start to eat. Or it may come on suddenly as they realize that they have eaten too much.

Interestingly, some people who have been binge eating for many years report that their sense of being out of control has faded over time, perhaps because experience has taught them that their binges are inevitable, so they no longer try to resist them. Some even plan ahead for what they see as unavoidable binges, thus setting up a self-fulfilling prophecy. Planning ahead allows these people to exercise some degree of control over when and where their binges take place, thereby minimizing their impact. They therefore feel that they have not lost control. This is not really the case, however, since they are still unable to prevent the episodes from occurring. Furthermore, many of these people report being unable to stop eating once they have started. This seems to be the case even when a binge is interrupted—say, the telephone may ring or someone may come to the door—as when this happens, it is common for the binge to be suspended only to restart once the interruption ends.

HOW PEOPLE BINGE

People vary widely in how often they binge and what foods they eat. It is therefore difficult to define a typical binge in these terms.

Frequency and Duration

To be given a diagnosis of the eating disorder bulimia nervosa or binge eating disorder, two of the three main eating disorders recognized in adults (see Chapter 2), a person's binges have to occur on average at least once a week. This threshold is arbitrary and has changed over the years. It has been criticized for implying that people who binge less frequently, or who do so intermittently, are less impaired, whereas this is often not the case. Consequently, clinicians often ignore thresholds of this type when making a diagnosis. What matters is whether the person has regular binges and whether their binges are interfering with their physical health or quality of life.

The significance of the frequency of binge eating is also confusing. If you binge "only once in a while," does this mean there is no need for concern? At what frequency is binge eating a problem? Is it the numbers—how often you binge, for how long, over what time span—that determine how serious the problem is? Or should the guiding factor be how much binge eating affects your life? As noted above, in practice clinicians are concerned with impairment—the degree to which binge eating interferes with physical health or quality of life.

How long do binges last? This depends on a variety of factors, a particularly important one being whether the person intends to vomit afterwards. Data from our patients in Oxford indicate that, among those who do vomit, binges last on average about an hour, whereas among those who do not, they are almost twice as long. This is almost certainly because those who vomit feel under pressure to complete their binge as soon as possible so that they can bring up the food and thereby minimize the amount absorbed.

The Foods Eaten in a Binge

The food I eat usually consists of my "forbidden" foods: chocolate, cake, cookies, jam, condensed milk, cereal, and improvised sweet food like raw cake mixture. Food that is easy to eat. Food that doesn't need any preparation. I never eat these kinds of food

*normally because they are so fattening. But when I binge I can't get
enough of them.*

When people who binge are asked "What do you eat when you binge?"
they typically give two types of reply. The first relates to the character
of the food. So they may reply "sweet
food" or "filling food." The second reply
relates to their attitude toward the food.
So they may answer "forbidden food,"
"dangerous food," or "fattening food."
What is clear is that most binges are composed of foods that the person is trying to avoid. This is a crucial point that we will return to
later. It is central to understanding the cause of many binges, and it is
central to overcoming binge eating and remaining well.

> *Most binges are composed
> of foods that the person
> is trying to avoid.*

You may have read that binges are characterized by their high
carbohydrate content and are driven by "carbohydrate craving"—a
widespread myth. In fact, the
proportion of carbohydrates in
binges is not particularly high,
no higher than that in ordinary meals. What characterizes
binges is not their composition in terms of carbohydrates, fats, and
proteins, but rather the overall amount eaten. If you binge or know
someone who does, you know that binges typically include cakes,
cookies, chocolate, ice cream, and so on. But, as Timothy Walsh of
Columbia University has pointed out, while it is commonly believed
that these foods are high in carbohydrates, they are more accurately
described as sweet foods with a high fat content.

> *Despite being a popular belief
> and a memorable phrase,
> "carbohydrate craving" is a myth.*

Interestingly, though, the notion of carbohydrate craving may
have had more relevance a decade or so ago. It is my impression
that the composition of binges changes over time and that it is governed by what foods are currently avoided or viewed as "forbidden."
Carbohydrates used to be regarded as "bad" foods and therefore fea-
tured prominently in binges, whereas more recently fats have had
the bad press. (Dietary fashions and fads are discussed in Chapter 5;
see p. 69.)

Figure 1 shows the eating record of someone with bulimia nervosa. It illustrates the typical eating pattern comprising undereating punctuated by episodes of binge eating.

The Size of Binges

The amount of food eaten during binges varies widely from person to person. Some people consume vast quantities of food; occasionally a person describes eating 15,000 to 20,000 calories at one time. However, this is not typical. When people are asked to describe exactly what they have eaten and then the number of calories is calculated, a typical binge contains between 1,000 and 2,000 calories. About a quarter of binges contain more than 2,000 calories which is close to the average daily calorie needs of many women (see Table 5, p. 70).

Laboratory studies support these accounts as similar figures have been obtained when people have volunteered to binge and then the precise composition of their binges has been calculated. One study found that one in every five patients with bulimia nervosa had binges of more than 5,000 calories and one in ten had binges of more than 6,000 calories.

While many binges are large, it is equally clear that many otherwise typical binges are small in size in that only average or even small amounts of food are consumed. These binges do not meet the technical definition of a binge described earlier owing to their small size, yet the person views them as binges because the amount eaten is perceived as excessive and there is an accompanying sense of loss of control. The Eating Disorder Examination, an interview for assessing the features of eating disorders that I devised together with my colleague Zafra Cooper, describes such binges as *subjective binges*. In contrast, binges in which truly large amounts are eaten are referred to as *objective binges*.

Subjective binges are not uncommon and can be a cause of considerable distress. They are especially typical of people who are attempting to adhere to a strict diet, including those with the eating disorder

Subjective binges are not uncommon and can be a cause of considerable distress.

Day _Tuesday_ Date _June 18th_

Time	Food and drink consumed	Place	*	V/L	Context and comments
6:30	Black coffee Glass of water	Bedroom			Sleepless night. Feel gross and fat.
11:45	Black coffee 2 glasses of water	Staff room			Will not binge today! Starting to feel hungry so had an extra glass of water.
2:15	1 medium bottle diet coke ½ donut	Staff room			Ohh! Why do they ALWAYS have donuts? Only had half though, so it's OK.
3:30	4 donuts	Staff bathroom	*		Why do I do this? Couldn't help myself but did not want anyone to see me. Feel horrible and fat.
6:15	1 medium bottle of diet coke Glass of water	Kitchen			Am not going to eat again today.
9:30	Pita bread and hummus	Bedroom	*		Am disgusted with myself. I have no willpower. Feel desperately alone.
	3 cinnamon raisin bagels		*		
	6 spoons of peanut butter		*		
	15 Oreo cookies		*	V	
	½ gallon vanilla ice cream		*		
	3 handfuls of nuts Large bottle of diet coke		*	V	Going to bed early to stop any further eating.

FIGURE 1. An eating record of someone with bulimia nervosa. Note the undereating in the first half of the day followed by binge eating later on. (Asterisks signify eating viewed by the person as excessive. V/L signifies vomiting or laxative use.)

anorexia nervosa. (In Chapter 2 I describe the various "eating disorders.")

The Cost of Binges

> *Spending on food is my biggest single expense every month. Over the years it's got me further and further into debt.*

Binge eating can be expensive and can get people into financial difficulties. This explains in part why some people resort to stealing food. Figure 2 illustrates the cost of binge eating. Scott Crow and colleagues in Minneapolis recently studied the monetary cost of binge eating in a sample of people with bulimia nervosa. They found that about a third of people's food bills were accounted for by the food that they consumed during their binges.

ARE ALL BINGES THE SAME?

Binges vary considerably, not only from person to person but also within a single individual. It is common for people to report that they have more than one type of binge, although some of these binges may not fit the technical definition (of an objective binge). One person described having three types of binge.

Full-Blown Binges

> *I eat and I eat, usually very fast, and without enjoyment, apart from initial taste pleasure which anyway is tempered with guilt. Usually furtively, and in one place: at home, the kitchen; at college, my room. I eat until I physically cannot eat any more. This is usually the type of binge where I take laxatives—during and after—which intensifies the feeling of panic and guilt. Immediately afterwards I am so physically bloated that emotions are dulled, but later I feel terrible.*

```
Please Check Your Bags Before Leaving
   No Refunds Without This Receipt
******** Your Purchases Today ********
        KELLOGGS CORN PUPS      3.69 F
        BTZIOS PIZZA            5.99 F
        NABISCO OREO            3.49 F
Regular Price 4.49 , You saved 1.00
        BRYRS ICE CR      PC    6.99 F
    1 @ 2/5.00
        PETER PAN PNUT BTT      2.50 F
Regular Price 3.49 , You saved 0.99
        THOMAS NY BAGEL         3.49 F
Regular Price 4.49 , You saved 1.00
        M&M PEANUT 8.2OZ        3.19 B
        BH GOUDA CHEESE         5.99 F
        DIET COKE 1.25L         1.19 B
   DP   SINGLE DEPOSIT          0.05 F
        MURRAY S/F COOKIES      3.49 F
        TAX                     0.36

   **** BALANCE               40.42
```

FIGURE 2. The cost of binge eating: a supermarket receipt showing the cost (in U.S. dollars) of the food bought for a single binge.

Half-Binges

These usually take place late at night and are similar to full-blown binges except that I eat food hurriedly in one place, and without enjoyment, but also without a great deal of panic. It is almost an automatic reaction, often to some situation. I can stop these.

Slow-Motion Binges

Usually I have these at home, not college. I can see them coming in advance. I may fight them for a while, but eventually I give in and *have an almost pleasurable feeling. There's definitely a release of ten-sion at the time because I don't have to worry anymore. I actually enjoy these binges, at least to start with. I choose foods that I like and don't usually allow myself or allow myself only in limited quantities. I may spend time preparing the food. At some stage it hits me what a fool I'm being and how much weight I will gain (not how greedy I am being), and then I become even more guilty, but I still feel a compulsion to carry on.*

Certain groups of people have distinctive binges. For example, people with the eating disorder anorexia nervosa often have small, subjective binges, but these are accompanied by the same distress and sense of loss of control that is associated with objective binges. And the binges of people who are significantly overweight (many of whom have "binge eating disorder"; see Chapter 2) tend not to be distinct in the sense that their beginning and end can be difficult to identify. These binges generally last longer than those of people with bulimia nervosa; indeed, they can last almost all day.

HOW BINGES BEGIN

By now you may be baffled by the fact that binge eating occurs at all. Why would something that leaves people feeling disgusted and ashamed happen again and again? This raises two issues. What causes binge eating problems to begin in the first place, and what keeps them going? These matters are addressed in Chapter 6. Also important, however, are the more immediate triggers of individual binges. What circumstances tend to precipitate a binge?

Many things trigger binges. A classic early study identified the main triggers of binges and a more recent one obtained information on exactly where they take place (see Box 1). Some of the most common triggers are described in the following paragraphs.

Undereating and the Associated Hunger. Some people who binge, especially those with bulimia nervosa or anorexia nervosa, eat

---

BOX 1. The triggers of binges and where they take place.

A detailed description was obtained of the binges of 32 patients seen at an eating disorder clinic in Sydney, Australia.[1] The majority met diagnostic criteria for bulimia nervosa (see Chapter 2). The main precipitants of their binges were reported to be as follows:

91%	Tension
84%	Eating something (anything at all)
78%	Being alone
78%	Craving specific foods
75%	Thinking of food
72%	Going home (either after school or work)
59%	Feeling bored and lonely

Thirty-three women with binge eating disorder (see Chapter 2) were given handheld computers for a week.[2] At regular intervals they were asked questions about their eating and mood. It emerged that their binges most commonly occurred when they were alone and in the following places:

31%	Kitchen
31%	Living room
10%	Car
10%	At work

---

[1]*Source:* Abraham, S. F., & Beumont, P. J. V. (1982). How patients describe bulimia or binge eating. *Psychological Medicine, 12,* 625–635.

[2]*Source:* Stein, R. I., Kenardy, J., Wiseman, C. V., Dounchis, J. Z., Arnow, B. A., & Wilfley, D. E. (2007). What is driving the binge in binge eating disorder? *International Journal of Eating Disorders, 40,* 195–203.

little outside their binges. The resulting deprivation can have many undesirable effects, as it would for anyone who was essentially starving him- or herself. Imposing strict limits on eating and eating too little creates a mounting physiological and psychological pressure to eat, and once eating starts it can be difficult to stop. Many say that it is like a dam bursting.

The urge to binge usually begins around midday on a "normal" day—that is, a day on which I am trying not to eat. During the afternoon thoughts of food become more and more of a preoccupation; and eventually at around 4:00 P.M. my power of concentration will be sufficiently nonexistent for thoughts about food to be totally overwhelming. So I leave work and go to the store.

One thing that definitely sets me off is hunger. If I am hungry, instead of eating something to satisfy it, I eat anything I can lay my hands on. It's almost as if I have to satisfy all tastes, even for things I don't like.

Breaking a Dietary Rule. Many people who binge also diet, and their dieting tends to be highly characteristic in its form (as we will discuss in Chapter 4). They are usually trying to follow strict rules about what, when, and how much they should eat. Breaking such rules commonly triggers a binge.

Drinking Alcohol. Some people find that drinking alcohol makes them vulnerable to binge. There are a number of reasons for this link. Alcohol reduces the ability to resist immediate desires and so interferes with the ability to stick to dietary rules. For example, a plan to eat only a salad could, after a few drinks, be readily abandoned in favor of eating a full meal. Alcohol also impairs judgment and causes people to underestimate how bad they will feel if they break their rules. In addition, alcohol makes some people feel gloomy and depressed, thereby further increasing the risk of binge eating.

Unpleasant Emotions. Unpleasant feelings of all types can trigger binges. Feeling depressed is a particularly powerful stimulus.

Binges start when I'm tired or depressed or just upset. I become tense and panicky and feel very empty. I try to block out the urge to eat, but it just grows stronger and stronger. The only way to release these feelings is to binge. And binge eating does numb feelings. It blots out whatever it was that was upsetting me. The trouble is that it is replaced with feeling guilty, self-critical, and drained.

Other emotional triggers include stress, tension, hopelessness, loneliness, boredom, irritability, anger, and anxiety.

Unstructured Time. The absence of structure in the day makes some people prone to binge, whereas having a routine may be protective. Lack of structure may also be accompanied by feelings of boredom, one of the moods that tend to trigger binge eating.

Being Alone. As already mentioned, binges mostly occur in secret. Being alone therefore increases the risk as there are no social constraints against binge eating. If the person is lonely as well, the risk is even greater.

Feeling Fat. Feeling fat is an experience reported by many women—it is uncommon in men—but the intensity and frequency of the "feeling" appear to be greater among those who have an eating problem. (I discuss feeling fat in more detail in Chapter 4.) In these people feeling fat tends to be equated with being fat, whatever the person's actual shape or weight. And feeling fat can trigger binge eating.

Gaining Weight. Most people who are concerned about their weight react badly to any increase. A weight gain as little as 1 pound (0.5 kilograms) may precipitate a negative reaction and, among those prone to binge, one response is to give up attempts to control eating with a binge being the result. This reaction is based upon a misunderstanding: body weight fluctuates within the day and from day to day, and short-term changes reflect changes in hydration not body fat. (In Chapter 5 I discuss body weight and weight fluctuations; and on p. 66 I provide advice on how to interpret the number on the scale.)

Premenstrual Tension. Some women report that they find it particularly difficult to control their eating in the few days before a menstrual period. This may be their response to various factors including feeling bloated, premenstrual weight gain, or to an adverse mood such as depression or irritability.

HOW BINGES END

After a binge I feel frightened and angry. Fear is a large part of what I feel. I am terrified about the weight I will gain. I also feel anger toward myself for allowing it to happen yet again. Binge eating makes me hate myself.

The hardest thing after a binge is waiting for the effects to die down. I hate feeling so useless and unable to do anything. Sometimes I feel I could literally rip open my stomach and pull out the garbage inside, the disgust and revulsion are so great. Failing that, laxatives are the next best thing.

After everyday overeating, most people either accept the episode as an indulgence ("naughty but nice") or have some feelings of guilt (more accurately they feel regret). They may decide to compensate by eating less and perhaps by exercising, but their self-recrimination and compensatory behavior are likely to end there.

The aftermath of binge eating is quite different. Those who binge often report that they experience some immediate, though temporary, positive feelings. For example, they may experience a sense of relief from the psychological and physiological deprivation that preceded it. Feelings of depression or anxiety that triggered the binge may also have dissipated. But these positive effects are soon replaced by feelings of shame, disgust, and guilt. Self-recrimination sets in, and people feel hopeless about ever being able to control their eating. Anxiety is also common as fears of weight gain mount. These negative feelings may be exacerbated by the physical effects of having binged, with sleepiness and abdominal distension being particularly common. The fear of weight gain may be so intense that it drives some people to take extreme compensatory measures which, ironically, may encourage yet further episodes of binge eating (as we will discuss in detail in Chapter 4).

CHAPTER 2

Eating Problems
and Eating Disorders

Few people have not heard of bulimia nervosa and the "dieter's disease" anorexia nervosa. Unfortunately the publicity that these disorders have attracted has resulted in them being trivialized; for example, the term *anorexic* is now synonymous with being underweight. One of the goals of this chapter is to clarify what these terms actually mean, while also explaining how binge eating problems are classified.

EATING PROBLEMS
VERSUS EATING DISORDERS

The great majority of people who binge do not have an "eating disorder." Their binge eating is occasional rather than frequent, it does them no physical harm, and it does not impair their quality of life. If, however, they view their binge eating as a "problem," then that is exactly what it is, an "eating problem." On the other hand, there are significant numbers of people whose binge eating does interfere with their physical health or quality of life. These people are viewed as having an eating disorder.

The great majority of people who binge do not have an "eating disorder."

In adults and teenagers three eating disorders are distinguished:

21

- Bulimia nervosa
- Anorexia nervosa
- Binge eating disorder

This is not the complete picture, however. Clinical and community-based studies indicate that it is not uncommon for people to have an eating disorder that falls outside these three categories. These people may be viewed as having an "atypical eating disorder."

BULIMIA NERVOSA

Bulimia nervosa, originally known in North America as "bulimia," has come to attention only in the last 30 or so years. Box 2 lists the major milestones in the history of this "new" eating disorder.

In principle, three features have to be present to make the diagnosis bulimia nervosa, and one feature has to be absent. These features are as follows:

1. The person must have frequent objective binges; that is, he or she must have recurrent episodes of eating during which he or she eats genuinely large amounts of food—taking into account the circumstances—with there being a sense of loss of control at the time. By definition, all people with bulimia nervosa binge eat.
2. The person must engage in one or more extreme methods of weight control. These include self-induced vomiting, the misuse of laxatives or diuretics, intensive exercising, and extreme dieting or fasting.
3. The person must show "overevaluation" of the importance of his or her shape or weight, or both; that is, people with bulimia nervosa should judge themselves largely, or even exclusively, in terms of their ability to control their shape or weight. (This feature is described in detail in Chapter 4, p. 55.) Their concern about shape and weight goes far beyond just feeling fat or being unhappy with their appearance.

BOX 2. A brief history of bulimia nervosa.

1976—Reports of "bulimarexia" among American college students (see Chapter 3).

1979—Publication of Professor Gerald Russell's classic paper "Bulimia nervosa: An ominous variant of anorexia nervosa." This paper introduced the term *bulimia nervosa.*

1980—Syndrome of "bulimia" added to the American Psychiatric Association's diagnostic manual.

1980–1982—Studies in Great Britain and North America indicate that bulimia nervosa is likely to be common (see Chapter 3).

1981–1982—Reports describe two promising treatments for bulimia nervosa: cognitive behavior therapy and antidepressant medication (see Chapter 8).

1987—*Bulimia* redefined and renamed *bulimia nervosa* by the American Psychiatric Association, bringing the concept more in line with Russell's one.

2013—Diagnostic criteria of the American Psychiatric Association broadened to include cases in which the binge eating occurs once a week. Previously the lower limit was twice weekly.

---

4. The person does not currently have anorexia nervosa (defined shortly). In effect this means that the person cannot be significantly underweight. In practice the great majority of those with the three defining features of bulimia nervosa have a body weight in the healthy range. Figure 3 shows the weight distribution of people with bulimia nervosa, anorexia nervosa, and binge eating disorder.

As explained in Chapter 3, bulimia nervosa is largely confined to women, with the majority being in their 20s. The proportion of cases that are male is uncertain—it is likely to be less than one in

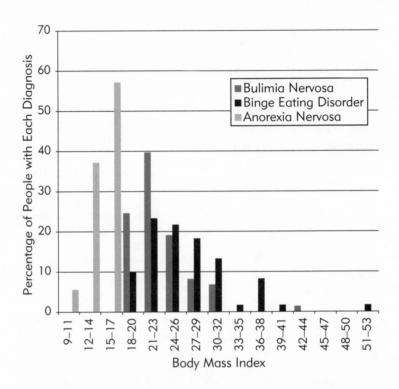

FIGURE 3. The weight distribution of people with bulimia nervosa, anorexia nervosa, and binge eating disorder (see p. 27) shown in terms of their body mass index (see Box 3). Data kindly provided by Dr. Riccardo Dalle Grave.

10. The problem usually starts in the late teenage years with a period of strict dieting that eventually becomes punctuated by repeated episodes of binge eating. In about a quarter of cases the dieting is so extreme that the person first develops anorexia nervosa and then progresses to bulimia nervosa.

People with bulimia nervosa have chaotic eating habits. All have objective binges, but these binges occur against the background of extreme attempts to restrict eating—indeed, the person's eating outside their binges closely resembles that of people with anorexia nervosa. Some eat virtually nothing outside their binges, and most of the others diet strictly. Many make themselves vomit after each binge in order to get rid of the food they have eaten. Laxatives, diuretics, and diet pills may also be used for this purpose, as may intense exercising.

Once established, bulimia nervosa tends to be self-perpetuating. It has little tendency to remit spontaneously, although it can wax and wane in severity. By the time people seek help, if indeed they do, most have eaten in this way for 5 to 10 years or even longer.

ANOREXIA NERVOSA

Most people have heard of anorexia nervosa, perhaps because of the media attention it attracts, either because it can be fatal or because the sufferers look so unwell. Two main conditions must be met for someone to be said to have this eating disorder:

1. The person should be significantly underweight, and this should be the result of his or her own efforts. The threshold for viewing someone as significantly underweight is debated and varies—a body mass index (BMI) below 17.5, 18.0, or 18.5 are widely used figures. (Box 3 describes the BMI.)
2. The person should show evidence of the overevaluation of the importance of shape and weight, as in bulimia nervosa. Rather than worrying about being underweight, people with anorexia nervosa are terrified of gaining weight and becoming fat. Indeed, many regard themselves as already being "fat" despite their low weight. For this reason they are sometimes said to have a "morbid fear of fatness" or a "weight phobia," and their dieting has been described as being driven by a "relentless pursuit of thinness."

Anorexia nervosa mainly affects teenage girls and young women, but about one in 10 cases occurs in men. People with the disorder achieve their low weight by eating very little, although excessive exercising may also contribute. They avoid eating foods they view as

---

BOX 3. The body mass index (BMI).

The body mass index (BMI) is a useful way of determining whether you are underweight, normal weight, or overweight. It is your weight adjusted for your height. Specifically it is weight in kilograms divided by height in meters squared (i.e., weight/[height × height]). The BMI applies to all adults of both sexes between the ages of 18 and 60. Appendix II provides a chart for identifying your BMI.

Below are the BMI thresholds used to classify people as underweight, as having a healthy weight, as overweight, or as having obesity. Note that they are based on health risks, not appearance.

Underweight	Below 18.5
Healthy weight	18.5 to 24.9
Overweight	25.0 to 29.9
Obese	30.0 and above

There is good evidence that people of Asian origin have greater health risks at lower BMIs than Caucasians. For this reason, the World Health Organization has considered lowering the BMI thresholds for overweight and obesity for Asian people.

It is also important to bear in mind that there are some limitations of the BMI. It does not apply to children below 18, adults above 60, people with a large muscle mass (e.g., many athletes), or those with physical illnesses.

---

fattening, and they may fast at times. About a third have "binges," most of which are small in size (i.e., they are subjective binges), during which their attempts to restrict their food intake break down. For people with anorexia nervosa a binge may consist simply of a few cookies.

> I had been anorexic for about a year and was attempting to start eating properly. One day, out of the blue, I ate a chocolate cookie. Suddenly I began eating all those things I'd deprived myself of. It wasn't a

large binge by my current standards, but it was more calories than I
normally ate in a whole week. I came out of my trance-like state and
was suddenly terrified about what I had done. I immediately went to
the bathroom and stuck my fingers down my throat. I had to throw
up and get rid of all the garbage inside me.

Anorexia nervosa may be short-lived with the person making a
complete recovery with or without treatment. This is most typical of
cases in their teens. Alternatively, it may evolve into bulimia nervosa
or an atypical eating disorder (see below). A small proportion of sufferers get "stuck" in anorexia nervosa, an extremely serious state from
which it can be hard to escape.

BINGE EATING DISORDER

As the term implies, binge eating is the main feature of binge eating disorder. The diagnosis is a recent one, although its origins go
back to the late 1950s when Albert Stunkard of the University of
Pennsylvania noted that some people with obesity have significant
problems with binge eating. This observation was largely ignored or
forgotten until the mid-to-late 1980s when evidence began to mount
that about a quarter of those who seek treatment for obesity report
binge eating, yet few meet the criteria for bulimia nervosa. About the
same time, community studies of the prevalence of bulimia nervosa
showed that the majority of those who binge eat do not have bulimia
nervosa. Together, these findings led to the proposal that a new eating disorder be recognized characterized by recurrent binge eating in
the absence of extreme methods of weight control. This disorder is
now termed *binge eating disorder*. Prior to this, such people had been
described, somewhat pejoratively, as "compulsive eaters."

People with binge eating disorder have repeated objective binges,
but they do not engage in the extreme weight control measures used
by people with bulimia nervosa. Thus they do not vomit; they do
not take laxatives, diuretics, or diet pills; they do not overexercise;

and they do not diet to an extreme degree. Instead, their eating is typically characterized by a general tendency to overeat upon which binge eating is superimposed. This is illustrated in the eating record shown in Figure 4. Hardly surprisingly, therefore, many people with binge eating disorder are overweight or have frank obesity (as shown in Figure 3).

Binge eating disorder affects a broader range of people than anorexia nervosa and bulimia nervosa; the gender distribution is more even with about a third of cases being male, and the age range is broader, stretching from the teens to middle age. It also tends to have a phasic course in which there are periods when the person is prone to binge interspersed with others when he or she has control over eating. These phases may be quite long, lasting months or even years.

Community-based studies of binge eating disorder indicate that those who seek help are an atypical subgroup. The cases in the community are younger and most are not overweight.

THE ATYPICAL EATING DISORDERS

Many eating disorders do not meet the diagnostic criteria for anorexia nervosa, bulimia nervosa, or binge eating disorder. These eating disorders have attracted a variety of labels, one of which used to be "eating disorder not otherwise specified" or "ED-NOS." In this book I will employ the less cumbersome term *atypical eating disorder*.

The atypical eating disorders are those eating disorders seen in adults and teenagers that do not fit the technical definitions of anorexia nervosa, bulimia nervosa, or binge eating disorder. The category has recently attracted considerable attention as it has been discovered that it is much more common than had been assumed (see Figure 5). In common with bulimia nervosa and anorexia nervosa, it mainly affects teenage girls and young women.

The atypical eating disorders may be divided into five more-or-less distinct subgroups:

Day _Thursday_   Date _April 20th_

Time	Food and drink consumed	Place	*	V/L	Context and comments
8:10	Plain bagel, butter Decaf	Kitchen			
8:25	Half bagel, butter Decaf	Kitchen	*		Great bagel, but . . .
10:20	1 raisin muffin Decaf	At desk			Thinking about eating all morning
12:00	Medium pizza— pepperoni Large diet coke	Staff cafeteria			Feel somewhat sick. Really full. I'm enormous.
3:00	2 donuts Decaf 2 donuts	At desk	* *		Must stop buying these. They are too good!
6:30	Large bag potato chips Diet coke 2 plain bagels with peanut butter Large slice chocolate cake Diet coke	Kitchen— standing	* * *		Tiresome drive home. Restless. I've nothing to do . . . just started eating . . . mindlessly. Enjoyed it at first.
7:15	3 KitKats Decaf tea 6 scoops chocolate ice cream 1 Cherry yogurt	Kitchen	* * *		I've started again. This is hopeless. I've no self-control.
9:00	2 decaf tea				

FIGURE 4. An eating record of someone with binge eating disorder.
Note the general tendency to overeat, upon which binge eating is superimposed.
(Asterisks signify eating viewed by the person as excessive. V/L signifies vomiting
or laxative use.)

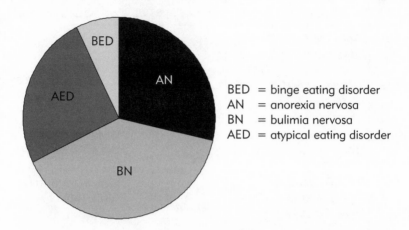

FIGURE 5. Pie chart showing the distribution of the four eating disorder diagnoses among adult patients attending a well-established eating disorder clinic. Data taken from Fairburn, C. G., & Cooper, Z. (2011). Eating disorders, DSM-5 and clinical reality. *British Journal of Psychiatry, 198,* 8–10.

1. *Subthreshold bulimia nervosa* in which the eating disorder resembles bulimia nervosa but just fails to meet its diagnostic criteria.

2. *Subthreshold anorexia nervosa* in which the eating disorder resembles anorexia nervosa but just fails to meet its diagnostic criteria.

3. *Subthreshold binge eating disorder* in which the eating disorder resembles binge eating disorder but just fails to meet its diagnostic criteria.

4. *Mixed eating disorders* in which the features of bulimia nervosa, anorexia nervosa, or binge eating disorder are combined in such a way as to make it impossible to classify the state as a variant of a single one of these disorders.

5. *Night eating syndrome* in which there are recurrent episodes of eating in the evening or during the night.

MIXED EATING DISORDERS

What may be termed *mixed eating disorders* are the most common form of atypical eating disorder. The term refers to eating disorders in which the features of anorexia nervosa and bulimia nervosa, and sometimes binge eating disorder, are jumbled up together. An example would be someone with the overevaluation of shape and weight that is characteristic of anorexia nervosa and bulimia nervosa, a somewhat low weight (but not low enough to be said to have anorexia nervosa), occasional but not regular binges, extreme dieting, and intermittent self-induced vomiting.

What is known about such eating disorders is that they are equivalent to bulimia nervosa in terms of their severity, duration, and impact on the person's quality of life. Often the person has had anorexia nervosa or bulimia nervosa in the past. Binge eating is a common feature of the mixed eating disorders.

You may come across the term *purging disorder*. This is a term used by some clinicians to refer to an eating disorder in which there is recurrent purging (mainly in the form of self-induced vomiting or the misuse of laxatives or diuretics) in the absence of binge eating. Our data from Oxford indicate that most of these people report having subjective binges and so may be better viewed as having a form of subthreshold bulimia nervosa.

NIGHT EATING SYNDROME

Night eating syndrome is a relatively new diagnosis about which much remains to be learned. In principle, three features have to be present to make the diagnosis:

1. Recurrent episodes of eating at night (after falling asleep) or eating excessively during the evening.
2. Awareness of the behavior at the time.
3. The pattern of eating results in significant distress or impairment.

Night eating syndrome tends to begin during early adulthood and it seems to run a long-term course, although there may be extended periods when it is not present. It tends to be particularly prevalent among people with insomnia or obesity and those with binge eating disorder. It appears to run in families, and it is equally common among men and women.

The only eating disorder that can get confused with night eating syndrome is binge eating disorder. There are four main differentiating features. In night eating syndrome the episodes of overeating only occur in the evening or at night; the episodes are relatively small in size (averaging about 300 calories); there is often no sense of loss of control at the time; and the eating is frequently motivated by the goal of getting back to sleep.

THE TRANSDIAGNOSTIC PERSPECTIVE

The diagnostic distinctions above delineate the main forms of eating disorders that exist. However, they have shortcomings. First, they can blind one to the important fact that people with eating disorders have a remarkable amount in common. Most important, they share similar eating habits and similar concerns about shape and weight. This results in some of the diagnostic distinctions being particularly difficult to make. Take, for example, a person with all the features of bulimia nervosa but a somewhat low weight—perhaps a BMI around 18.0. What diagnosis this person is given depends largely on whether this BMI is viewed as "significantly low"—a matter of debate. If it is viewed as significantly low, then they are likely to be given the diagnosis of anorexia nervosa; if it is not, the person will be said to have bulimia nervosa. Another problematic boundary is that between bulimia nervosa and binge eating disorder. In people who do not vomit or take laxatives, the distinction hinges mainly on how little they eat between their binges. If it is very little, they are likely to be given a diagnosis of bulimia nervosa, whereas if it is somewhat larger, they will be said to have binge eating disorder. In other words, there are no sharp dividing lines between the various eating disorders.

A second limitation of the diagnostic system is that the three eating disorder diagnoses provide an incomplete picture of the range of problems that are present, both in community and clinic samples. As we have already discussed, many eating disorders do not meet the diagnostic criteria for anorexia nervosa, bulimia nervosa, or binge eating disorder, and so have to be placed into a neglected residual category, termed here *atypical eating disorder*.

The meaningfulness of the diagnostic distinctions is further undermined by the fact that most eating disorders change in form over time. It is not uncommon for a person to be eligible for one eating disorder diagnosis in January and another in June, without a major change in their state. "Diagnostic migration" is the norm, rather than the exception. In my clinical practice I have encountered innumerable people in their 20s or 30s who have had an eating disorder since their teens, but at one stage it would have been called anorexia nervosa, later on bulimia nervosa, and most recently an atypical eating disorder. Have they really had three separate mental health disorders, one after the other? No, they have had a single eating problem that has evolved in form over time.

This book adopts a "transdiagnostic" perspective on eating problems and how to overcome them. Part I describes the full range of problems that people experience and what causes them to persist. Part II describes a way of breaking out of those eating problems in which binge eating is a major feature, irrespective of the eating disorder diagnosis.

CHAPTER 3

Who Binges?

For anyone who binges, the answer to this question is of great interest because many people have the sense that they are the only one. To a large extent this is the result of the shame and secrecy that accompany the behavior. This secrecy has been a problem for researchers too as it has made it difficult to discover exactly who does binge.

THE EMERGENCE OF BULIMIA NERVOSA

Interest in the number of people who binge has its origins in the identification of bulimia nervosa in the mid-1970s. The first sign of the problem came with the publication of a number of reports describing "bulimarexia" or the "binge–purge syndrome" among female students on U.S. college campuses. The problem came to wider attention with the publication in 1979 of a paper titled "Bulimia nervosa: An ominous variant of anorexia nervosa" written by Gerald Russell from London, a respected authority on anorexia nervosa. In this paper he described the characteristics of 30 patients (28 women and two men) whom he had seen between 1972 and 1978. These patients had bulimia nervosa as we know it today.

Simultaneously in Edinburgh, I was seeing a similar group of patients. The most striking thing about these patients was that the majority thought they were the only person with their type of eating problem. They thought that they alone had repeated bouts of uncontrolled overeating followed by vomiting or taking laxatives. Their view was not surprising since bulimia nervosa had not yet attracted public attention. Indeed, in those days binge eating had hardly been heard of.

Most of my Edinburgh patients had kept their eating problem secret for many years. They had done this in part because of shame and self-disgust and in part because they thought that nothing could be done to help them. And keeping the problem hidden was not too difficult since most had an unremarkable body weight and most could eat relatively normally when with others. Their binge eating occurred in private. Some described having eventually summoned up the courage to see their family doctor, only to be told that they could not have an eating problem because their weight was normal.

The fact that my patients had kept their problem hidden for many years suggested that it might not be an unusual variant of anorexia nervosa, as suggested by Gerald Russell; rather, it might be a significant health problem in its own right. The challenge was to find out whether this was indeed the case. How could hidden cases be uncovered?

The solution was to enlist the help of the magazine *Cosmopolitan*. Since most of my patients were young women, I guessed that many might read this magazine. So I arranged for a small notice to be placed in the April 1980 issue of the U.K. edition (see Figure 6). The result was dramatic. Within a week or so I had received letters from more than a thousand women, the majority of whom seemed certain to have bulimia nervosa (see Box 4).

More or less simultaneously in Chicago, Craig Johnson was receiving large numbers of requests for information following the publication of various popular articles on bulimia nervosa. He and his colleagues also sent out a number of questionnaires and in this way identified 361 women with bulimia nervosa (termed *bulimia* in the United States at the time). These women were very similar to those identified through *Cosmopolitan* (see Table 1).

Other clinics were also encountering cases of this "new" eating

New eating pattern

Some psychiatrists have become concerned recently over what may be the emergence of a new and bizarre eating disorder affecting young women in their late teens and twenties. The principal features are frequent self-induced and secretive vomiting and a profound fear of becoming fat.

The sufferers have an irresistible desire to eat and drink, but keep their weight normal by vomiting.

The condition is difficult to treat—and many GPs may not be fully acquainted with the symptoms and dangers—but even in a mild form it can have serious physical and psychological repercussions.

Psychiatrists would like to know more about the prevalence of the disorder. Anyone with experience of vomiting this way might be able to help research by answering a confidential questionaire. Write to: Dr C G Fairburn, University Department of Psychiatry, Royal Edinburgh Hospital, Morningside Park, Edinburgh EH10 5HF.

FIGURE 6. The *Cosmopolitan* notice (from the "Health Reports" page of the April 1980 issue).

disorder. More or less simultaneously the disorder emerged in North America, the United Kingdom, Australia, and New Zealand.

Little is known about the origins of bulimia nervosa. It is possible that it was a source of undetected suffering years, decades, or even centuries before the disorder was recognized. Indeed, the experience of my Edinburgh patients and those who responded to the *Cosmopolitan* notice indicates that the disorder certainly went undetected at least for a time. This said, there are far fewer documented cases of binge eating and purging predating the mid-20th century than there are of individuals who have had anorexia nervosa. Overall, it seems unlikely that bulimia nervosa plagued young women for centuries before the disorder was recognized. But the question of why there was such a dramatic upsurge in the 1970s remains unanswered. Research into the causes of bulimia nervosa provides some clues (see Chapter 6).

BOX 4. The *Cosmopolitan* study.

To find out whether bulimia nervosa was a significant, yet undetected, health problem, a notice was placed in the Health Reports page of the April 1980 issue of the women's magazine *Cosmopolitan* (see Figure 6). It asked people who were using self-induced vomiting as a means of weight control to write in if they were willing to complete a confidential questionnaire. Vomiting was chosen as the feature for identifying potential cases since it is the least ambiguous of the core features of bulimia nervosa.

Within a week or so more than a thousand replies were received. The first 800 were sent a questionnaire designed to obtain information on weight, eating habits, and attitudes toward shape and weight. Six hundred and sixty-nine questionnaires (84%) were returned fully completed. On the basis of the responses it was clear that 499 of the respondents were highly likely to have bulimia nervosa.

All 499 cases were women (remember, it was a women's magazine). Their average age was 24 years, and two-thirds were in their 20s. Over three-quarters (83%) had a body weight within the healthy range for their age and height. In most cases the eating problem had started in their teenage years, and they had been binge eating, on average, for 5 years. A quarter (27%) reported that they were binge eating at least daily, and over half (56%) vomited daily. Nineteen percent abused laxatives.

The degree of distress reported by these women was extreme. Many wrote lengthy letters pleading for help. Two-thirds (68%) had clinically significant levels of depression and anxiety. Most expressed surprise and relief at knowing that they were not the only one with the problem.

Over half these women thought that they needed professional help, yet only 2.5% were receiving any form of treatment. Of those who wanted help, fewer than half (43%) had ever mentioned the problem to a health professional.

The findings of this study strongly suggested that bulimia nervosa was a significant, largely undetected problem.

Source: Fairburn, C. G., & Cooper, P. J. (1982). Self-induced vomiting and bulimia nervosa: An undetected problem. *British Medical Journal, 284,* 1153–1155.

TABLE 1. A comparison of the samples recruited in two early surveys of bulimia nervosa.

	British sample	American sample
Age (in years)	23.8	23.7
Marital status		
Married (%)	20.7	18.4
Binge eating[a]		
Age at onset (years)	18.4	18.1
Duration (years)	5.2	5.4
Frequency—at least daily (%)	27.2	50.0
Self-induced vomiting		
Frequency—at least daily (%)	56.1	45.7
Laxative misuse		
Regular misuse (%)	18.8	33.0
Weight[a]		
Normal weight	83.2	61.6
Ever overweight (%)	45.2	50.1
Menstrual disturbance (%)	46.6	50.7

Sources: British sample—Fairburn, C. G., & Cooper, P. J. (1982). Self-induced vomiting and bulimia nervosa: An undetected problem. *British Medical Journal, 284,* 1153–1155.

American sample—Johnson, C. L., Stuckey, M. K., Lewis, L. D., & Schwartz, D. M. (1983). A survey of 509 cases of self-reported bulimia. In P. L. Darby, P. E. Garfinkel, D. M. Garner, & D. V. Coscina (Eds.), *Anorexia nervosa: Recent developments in research.* New York: Alan Liss.

[a]Different definitions were used in the two studies.

THE MATTER OF DETECTION

You will perhaps have been struck by the fact that only 2.5% of those identified in the *Cosmopolitan* study were in treatment. Today far more people seek help, but typically this is after a significant delay. Why is this? There are many reasons:

1. As we have already discussed, binge eating problems are accompanied by feelings of shame and guilt. By seeking treat-

ment, sufferers run the risk of others finding out about their problem and the years of deceit and subterfuge that have been required to keep it secret.

2. Men may find it particularly difficult admitting to having a binge eating problem as these problems are widely viewed as being confined to women.

3. Some people feel they do not deserve help.

4. Some people think their eating problem is not severe enough to merit treatment.

5. Some people hope the problem will resolve of its own accord.

6. Others do not want help as they obtain some benefit from the problem. For example, it might help them cope with intense emotions (see Chapter 6) or it might provide them with an excuse for not performing well in some aspect of life (e.g., career, relationships).

7. There may be financial barriers to getting help. Sufferers may not have the financial resources or insurance needed to cover the cost of treatment. Shockingly, some insurance companies do not provide coverage for the treatment of the atypical eating disorders.

8. It can be difficult to tell health professionals. Prior health problems (e.g., menstrual irregularity; see Chapter 5) may have been a result of the eating problem, yet the health professional was kept in the dark about their likely cause.

The fact that only a small proportion of those with binge eating problems are getting professional help is disturbing because there are treatments capable of helping them. These include the self-help program in Part II of this book.

THE FINDINGS OF COMMUNITY STUDIES

Since 1980 there have been numerous studies of the prevalence of binge eating problems. Most have focused on Caucasian women between the ages of 14 and 40 as they are thought to be most at risk.

However, more and more studies are including men, a broader age range, and different ethnic groups.

The method used to detect cases is usually a simple question-naire, but such questionnaires tend to generate inflated estimates. More reliable are the studies in which people are interviewed. Inter-estingly, these studies have produced relatively consistent findings. It seems that bulimia nervosa affects between 1 and 2% of young adult women whereas binge eating disorder affects about 2 to 3% of both men and women and a much broader age range. These figures are noteworthy as binge eating problems impair both quality of life (see Chapter 4) and physical health (see Chapter 5).

There have also been studies of children. These have found that binge eating does occur in children, particularly among those who are overweight. In one sample of 112 overweight children, over 5% met the criteria for binge eating disorder.

STUDIES OF OTHER SOCIAL GROUPS

There have been few studies of ethnic groups other than Caucasians. This is regrettable because there is evidence that Asian Americans and Hispanic Americans are prone to develop binge eating prob-lems—indeed, some studies have suggested that they may be even more vulnerable.

Lower and middle income countries have also been neglected. This is largely because eating disorders have tended to be viewed as "culture-bound syndromes" of the West. This view is now outdated as more and more evidence accumulates that they occur across the globe. For example, bulimia nervosa and anorexia nervosa most cer-tainly occur in both high- and low-income Asian countries including Japan, China, India, and Malaysia. In the Arab world, eating prob-lems are also becoming a public health concern.

CHAPTER 4

Psychological and Social Aspects

Sometimes a binge is just a binge. It is an isolated behavior that, even if recurrent, is not associated with other problems. More often than not, though, binge eating is associated with other difficulties. You may, in fact, be reading this book because of these difficulties rather than the binge eating. The relationship between these problems and the binge eating is complex, and often vicious circles develop that are self-maintaining and difficult to break.

The goal of this chapter and the next is to describe the many problems and concerns associated with binge eating and to examine their possible contribution to binge eating problems. This chapter focuses on problems that can be described as psychological or social; physical problems are examined in Chapter 5.

DIETING

Many people who binge also diet to an extreme degree, or at least attempt to do so, the exception being people with binge eating disorder. Sustained dieting punctuated by episodes of binge eating is the eating pattern seen in bulimia nervosa and those cases of anorexia nervosa in which there are binges. In some cases little or nothing is eaten outside the binges. In binge eating disorder the eating pattern is different. There is a tendency to overeat in general on top of which is superimposed the binge eating. People with binge eating disorder do diet at times: indeed, it is common for them to alternate between periods of successful dieting, which may last for months at a time, and periods of overeating when they also binge. As a result, their body weight may change markedly from month to month and year to year.

It is common for people with bulimia nervosa to make the mistake of thinking that their dieting is simply their response to binge eating. While dieting is undoubtedly encouraged by binge eating, especially among those who are highly concerned about their shape and weight, dieting plays an important role in causing binge eating. For example, binge eating is much more likely to occur on days in which the person is dieting. This is illustrated in Figure 7 which shows dieting both encouraging binge eating and being a response to it. Both

> *Dieting plays an important role in causing binge eating.*

these processes are powerful and together they result in binge eating persisting month after month, year after year. When tackling a binge eating problem it is therefore crucial to address not only the binge eating but also any contributory dieting.

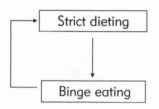

FIGURE 7. The vicious circle linking strict dieting and binge eating.

Three Forms of Dieting

There are three main ways in which people diet. People who binge, and particularly those with bulimia nervosa or anorexia nervosa, tend to practice all three of them.

Delaying Eating. Some people eat barely anything between their binges. Indeed, they may not eat for days at a time (i.e., they

fast). More commonly, though, they delay eating for as long as possible during the day, often not eating until the evening. About one
in four people with bulimia nervosa does this, whereas it is much
less common in binge eating disorder (about one in 20). Among the
general population, only about one in 100 does not eat during the
daytime.

Restricting the Overall Amount Eaten. Usually this involves
trying to keep food intake below a certain calorie limit. For many
people with bulimia nervosa the limit is 1,000 or 1,200 calories a day,
well below the amount needed for normal day-to-day functioning.
Some people set themselves even more extreme and inappropriate
calorie limits, such as 800 or even 600 calories a day.

Avoiding Certain Types of Food. People who binge may avoid
certain types of food because they perceive them as fattening or
because eating them has triggered binges in the past. They often
describe these foods as "forbidden," "bad," or "dangerous." Research
has shown that about one in five women in the general population
diets in this way. In contrast, three-quarters of those with bulimia
nervosa do so, as do half of those with binge eating disorder.

The range of foods avoided varies greatly. Among extreme dieters few foods—other than those manufactured and marketed as "diet
foods"—are eaten freely. Figure 8 shows the "avoided food list" of a
patient with bulimia nervosa.

It is not uncommon for those who diet strictly to describe what
they are doing as "healthy eating" or to justify their restrictive practices on the grounds that they are vegetarian or have a food allergy.
Whatever way dieting is described, any dietary restriction that is
intended at least in part to reduce weight or change shape should be
viewed as dieting.

The Effects of Dieting

*Food dominates my every waking minute. Even my dreams center
on food.*

Whole milk	Pancakes	Other pastas
Butter	Ice cream	Pizza
Cheese	Milkshakes	Fried chicken
Bread	Candy bars	French fries
Bagels	Soda	Chicken parm
Muffins	Potato chips	Ribs
Cereal	Tortilla chips	Meatloaf
Cookies	Salad dressing	Hotdogs
Cake	Mayonnaise	Hamburgers
Doughnuts	Macaroni salad	Chinese food
Peanut butter	Spaghetti/noodles	

FIGURE 8. A list of foods avoided by someone with bulimia nervosa.

Dieting has physical and psychological effects. The physical effects are described in Chapter 5. An important psychological effect is that the dieter becomes preoccupied with thoughts about food and eating and may also develop a sense of deprivation. Some dieters find themselves totally preoccupied with the very subject they are trying to avoid, unable to think about anything other than food and eating. They find it difficult to engage in everyday activities requiring concentration and even activities that demand minimal mental focus, such as watching television, may become impossible. No matter what they are doing, thoughts about food and eating keep intruding into their mind and even into their dreams. And as you may be aware if you have a friend or relative who is dieting, some also talk incessantly about food and eating. If you look at the figures in Table 2, you will see that preoccupation of this type is rare among young women in general, but as many as one in four of those with a binge eating problem is affected to a moderate or marked degree.

Strict versus Ordinary Dieting

The three forms of dieting just described are all *extreme*; that is, the restrictions on how much, what, and when the person eats are marked. The dieting of some people who binge, particularly those

TABLE 2. Preoccupation with thoughts about food and eating among women with binge eating problems and women in the general population.

	Women in the community (%)	Women with binge eating disorder (%)	Women with bulimia nervosa (%)
Little or none	95	57	49
Slight	3	18	23
Moderate	2	21	13
Marked	0	4	15

with bulimia nervosa, also tends to be *strict*. Rather than having a general goal, these people have a very specific one, and if they do not achieve it they feel they have failed. Most dieters might want to keep their calorie intake below, say, 1,500 calories a day and are likely to be content if they achieve this goal on more days than not. In contrast, strict dieters feel that they *must* achieve this goal to the letter and that they have "failed" if they eat any more than their "rules" allow.

> *Strict dieters who break a dietary rule are prone to "give up" temporarily and binge.*

When dieting is both extreme and strict, involving highly specific dietary rules that demand considerable restraint, repeated "failures" are likely. This is demoralizing. But to make matters worse, these failures trigger binges because strict dieters are prone to abandon dieting, at least temporarily, when they break their rules, and the result is a binge. This reflects their thinking style, one that is characteristic of many of those who binge, so-called "all-or-nothing" or "dichotomous" thinking. People with this type of thinking see things in extreme, or black-or-white, terms; they see themselves as succeeding or failing; they view foods as good or bad; and so on. As a result, dieting characterized by multiple strict rules and accompanied by all-or-nothing thinking create a cycle of binge eating and dieting, with each promoting the other.

OTHER MEANS OF CONTROLLING SHAPE
AND WEIGHT

Dieting is the most common weight control method practiced by those with binge eating problems. However, some utilize more extreme measures, including inducing vomiting and taking laxatives and diuretics. These forms of behavior are common in bulimia nervosa and anorexia nervosa and many atypical eating disorders but, by definition (as explained in Chapter 2), they are not present in binge eating disorder. Together, they are often referred to as "purging."

Self-Induced Vomiting

> I started vomiting after eating too much one day. It seemed a brilliant way to stay thin without dieting. I could eat as much as I wanted and then get rid of it. It would be so much easier than all that dieting.

> I eat until I literally cannot eat any more. Then, using my fingers I make myself sick. Over the next half hour, drinking water between vomits, I purge all the food from my stomach. I then feel despondent, depressed, alone, and desperately scared because I have lost control again. I feel physically terrible: exhausted, puffy-eyed, dizzy, weak, and my throat hurts. I am also scared because I know it is dangerous. After a couple of sessions of vomiting when I actually brought up blood, I tried to stop. But I continued to binge, and the fear that built up was so great that I started making myself sick again.

It is not widely known that as many as 5 to 10% of young women admit to having made themselves vomit, and as many as 2% of young adult women vomit as often as once or more a week. "Epidemics" of self-induced vomiting sometimes occur, for example, in college dorms. Self-induced vomiting is especially common among people with bulimia nervosa, but it also occurs in up to half of those with anorexia nervosa. While most of these people vomit to get rid of food they have eaten—that is, in an effort to limit the number of calories absorbed—over time other motives may be acquired; for example, some people find that vomiting releases tension.

Self-induced vomiting is not necessarily evidence of an eating disorder (as defined in Chapter 2). The key issue is whether the vomiting and the other features of the eating problem interfere with physical health or quality of life. A particularly important matter is whether the person has control over the behavior. If someone chooses to vomit on occasions, however socially unorthodox it might be, the behavior is unlikely to be evidence of an eating disorder. But if the vomiting is frequent or cannot be resisted, it is almost certainly indicative of a significant eating problem.

> I stop eating when I begin to feel ill. By then I have an overwhelming desire to rid myself of all the food I have eaten. I push my fingers down my throat and vomit again and again until I feel completely empty. This makes me feel relieved and cleansed. It also leaves me exhausted.

Usually self-induced vomiting is achieved by sticking an object down to the back of the throat to induce the gag reflex. After a while, however, some people can regurgitate at will by bending over and perhaps pressing on their stomach. There are others who cannot make themselves vomit, however hard they try.

Most people vomit after eating truly large amounts of food, but some people vomit after eating almost anything, particularly if they view it as fattening. Some people vomit just once after eating, and this rids them of sufficient food to relieve their anxiety over what they have eaten. Others vomit again and again until they cannot bring up anything more. This process can take an hour or more, and may leave them physically drained. A minority practice a flushing technique: They drink something, then vomit, drink again and vomit, drink again, and so on, repeating this process until the liquid comes back clear of any food. Only at this point do they feel confident that they have retrieved everything that they can. This practice is physically hazardous as it can result in electrolyte disturbance (see Chapter 5, p. 75).

The belief that vomiting is an effective means of getting rid of food is a mistaken one. While it clearly removes some of the food, laboratory studies have shown that it retrieves only about half the calories consumed. For example, one study found that while volunteers' binges averaged 2,131 calories, their vomit only comprised 979 calories.

Vomiting retrieves about half the calories consumed.

The relative ineffectiveness of vomiting explains why most people with bulimia nervosa are a normal weight. It is because they are living off the residue of each of their binges, the 50% they cannot retrieve. And remember the average binge contains between 1,000 and 2,000 calories (see p. 12).

Some people say that they know that they bring almost everything up when they vomit. This is usually because they eat a "marker" food (such as tomatoes) at the beginning of each binge and they repeatedly vomit until this food (i.e., the tomato skins) reappears. They are acting on the erroneous (geological) assumption that food is deposited in the stomach in layers. In fact, the stomach contents are churned around, so the reappearance of the marker food does not indicate that the stomach has been emptied of everything that has been eaten.

> I first started vomiting as a way of eating what I liked, without feeling guilty and without putting on weight. Vomiting was surprisingly easy and I was pretty pleased with myself. It was only later that I realized what a problem it had become.

> Over the past 8 years I have repeatedly said to myself: "This is going to be the last time that I throw up." At first I was not that bothered: I thought I could control it if I chose to. But it soon became clear that it had control over me. Now stopping seems completely beyond my reach.

If you take a long-term perspective, self-induced vomiting becomes even less attractive as a means of weight control. People who induce vomiting often describe the delight that they experienced when they first made themselves sick. Here was the answer to their problems: instead of struggling to control their urges to eat, they could give in yet not gain weight. In practice, they pay a heavy price because vomiting encourages overeating. This is the result of two mechanisms. First, since people believe that by vomiting they will avoid absorbing most of what they have eaten, their attempts to resist eating are undermined and as a result they tend to become more prone to binge, and furthermore their binges become larger in size. They also find that it is easier to vomit if their stomach is full. As a result of these processes a further vicious circle becomes established with vomiting being both a response to binge eating and a behavior that encourages it (see Figure 9). Indeed, vomiting can become one of the main processes that maintains binge eating. This is illustrated by the fact that many people who vomit are able to resist binge eating—which would otherwise be outside their control—if they know that there will be no opportunity to vomit.

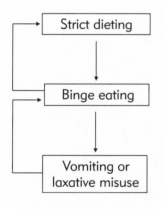

FIGURE 9. The vicious circles linking strict dieting, binge eating, and vomiting.

The one other point to stress is an obvious one. Vomiting has harmful physical effects. These are described in Chapter 5. Table 3 summarizes the key facts about self-induced vomiting.

TABLE 3. Four key facts about self-induced vomiting.

1. Vomiting is inefficient. It only retrieves about half the calories eaten in a typical binge.

2. Vomiting encourages overeating: people become more prone to binge and their binges become larger.

3. Vomiting maintains binge eating.

4. Vomiting has harmful physical effects.

Laxative and Diuretic Misuse

I started taking laxatives because I was scared that because I was eating so much I would get fat really quickly. I thought that if I took laxatives all the food would go straight through me.

I read in a magazine about people using laxatives as a way of purging themselves. I'd tried vomiting but couldn't do it. So I went out and bought some laxatives and downed 10 after every binge. I knew deep down that they didn't really do anything to counteract the binge, but they made me feel empty and cleansed inside.

The use of laxatives or diuretics (water pills) to control weight is less common than the use of self-induced vomiting. Laxatives are taken by about a third of those with bulimia nervosa and diuretics by about 10% (see Table 4). Both may occur in isolation or in combination with self-induced vomiting. By definition, all three forms of behavior are uncommon among those with binge eating disorder, although they do occur in anorexia nervosa and some atypical eating disorders.

People with binge eating problems misuse laxatives in two ways. They take them either to compensate for specific episodes of overeating, in which case the behavior is very similar to self-induced vomiting and the numbers taken may be very large, or they take them on a regular basis, independent of particular episodes of overeating, in which case the number taken is smaller and the behavior is more like dieting. Diuretics tend to be taken in the latter way.

Laxatives have little effect on calorie absorption because most food is absorbed high up in the intestine whereas laxatives act lower down. Diuretics have no effect on calorie absorption: they are merely dehydrating. Nevertheless some people find the use of these drugs rewarding, mainly because weight drops, albeit transitorily, due to the fluid lost in the diarrhea or excess urine. (In Chapter 5, p. 66, I discuss hydration and its importance in relation to body weight.) In addition, some people find that taking laxatives gives them a sense of having rid themselves, or "cleansed" themselves, of the food that they have eaten. In this way laxatives, like self-induced vomiting, can encourage further binge eating. Many people also describe liking the feeling that their abdomen is empty after taking laxatives, and some particularly value the flat appearance that may temporarily result. A minority welcome the unpleasant physical effects. They view the abdominal cramps and spasms, and the associated diarrhea, as just punishment for having overeaten.

The physical effects of laxative and diuretic misuse are described in Chapter 5.

Diet Pills

Diet pills, typically appetite suppressants, are also misused by some of those with eating disorders. This is despite the fact that these drugs only have a modest effect on body weight.

TABLE 4. Common methods of weight control (besides dieting) in people with bulimia nervosa.

	Community sample (%)	Clinic sample (%)
Self-induced vomiting	54	76
Laxative misuse	35	38
Both vomiting and laxative misuse	19	23
Diuretic misuse	10	12

Extreme Exercising

Some people who binge exercise a lot, in large part to influence their shape or weight. This is not usually a problem unless it starts to take over their life. If it begins to take precedence over other important activities, such as eating, sleeping, or socializing, it is of greater concern.

A subset of people develop driven or "compulsive" exercising. This is characterized by difficulty resisting exercising, even when the costs far outweigh the benefits, and it is most often seen in anorexia nervosa. In these people "overuse injuries" may occur.

Another exercise-related phenomenon is "debting." This is when eating and exercising become linked in such a way that the people will not eat unless they have burned off the requisite number of calories beforehand. It tends to coexist with extreme exercising and, although unusual, it is seen in all the eating disorders other than binge eating disorder.

At the other end of the spectrum, exercising too little is more characteristic of people with obesity including those with binge eating disorder. This contributes both to their obesity and to its associated health risks.

Manipulation of Fluid Intake

It is not uncommon for people who binge to manipulate their fluid intake as a means of controlling their eating or weight. Among the behaviors seen are the following:

- Drinking large quantities of fluid in order to curb appetite and feel full.
- Drinking large quantities of fluid to facilitate vomiting.
- "Flushing"—after binge eating, repeated drinking followed by vomiting until the liquid comes back clear of any food.
- Minimizing fluid intake in order to dehydrate (and lose weight).

All of these behaviors can disturb the body's level of hydration and electrolyte levels too (as we shall discuss in Chapter 5, p. 75).

PHYSICAL AND PSYCHOLOGICAL EFFECTS OF BEING UNDERWEIGHT

Some people with binge eating problems are unambiguously underweight, even if they do not view themselves this way. Anyone with a BMI of 18.5 or below is underweight medically speaking (see Chapter 2, p. 26) and is at risk of adverse physical, psychological, and social effects. These markedly increase once the BMI falls below 17.5.

Knowledge about the consequences of a low body weight has come from a variety of sources. These include studies of the effects of famines and experimental studies in which volunteers have adhered to a restricted diet for extended periods of time, the most famous being the Minnesota Semi-Starvation Study (see Box 5). Consistent findings have emerged from these studies and they are summarized below. If you are underweight and have an eating disorder you will experience the same effects, some of which are due to being underweight whereas others are direct effects of undereating. Almost all these effects are reversed by gaining weight to a healthy level and eating well.

Psychological Effects

Thinking. The brain is affected by both undereating and being underweight. It is therefore hardly surprising that thinking is impaired. It becomes somewhat inflexible, with there being difficulty switching from topic to topic. Decision making is also affected, and this often results in procrastination.

Concentration is almost always impaired although some people are unaware of this since they force themselves to focus on what they are doing. The concentration impairment is worsened by the presence of intrusive thoughts about food and eating.

BOX 5. The Minnesota semi-starvation study.

A seminal study of the effects of being underweight was conducted in the 1940s by Ancel Keys of the University of Minnesota. In this study 36 conscientious objectors (all male) were observed and assessed while their food intake was decreased to the point where their weight dropped to 75% of their prestarvation weight. The selection criteria for the men were strict: only the most socially and physically healthy volunteers were allowed to take part. Despite this, during the starvation period it was noticed that the once gregarious men became inward looking; they lost interest in socializing and other activities; and they became much more irritable, often provoking fights with each other. The men began to focus their lives around food and eating, paying little attention to anything else. This is very like what is seen in anorexia nervosa.

Source: Keys, A., Brozek, J., Henschel, A., Mickelsen, O., & Taylor, H. L. (1950). *The biology of human starvation* (2 vols.). Minneapolis: University of Minnesota Press.

The almost constant thinking about food and eating has secondary effects. It leads some people to become particularly interested in cooking and thus they selectively read recipes and watch TV cooking shows. They may also do a lot of cooking themselves. They may even take up careers that involve food and eating. A consequence of this focus on food and eating is that they become less interested in other things—for example, they may abandon prior interests and hobbies.

Emotions. Mood is affected by being underweight. It is generally somewhat low and many people are prone to get irritated rather easily.

Behavior. There are also remarkably consistent changes in behavior. One of the most prominent behavioral changes is heightened "obsessiveness." This term refers to the tendency to be inflexible and rigid in one's routines, and it is often accompanied by difficulty being spontaneous. The obsessiveness is particularly striking when it comes to eating, which may become a mini "ceremony" that has to be conducted alone. Some people eat very slowly, chewing each mouthful a certain number of times; others eat in a ritualized way, such as always eating from a certain plate or cutting food into small pieces. Hoarding objects is yet another sign of the obsessiveness although not everyone shows it. The hoarding may be of food or other things. Often people cannot explain why they are hoarding.

Social Effects

Being underweight has a profound effect on social functioning. There is a tendency to become inward-looking and self-focused. This is exaggerated by the heightened need for routine and predictability, and the difficulty being spontaneous. As a result people often withdraw socially and get used to this way of living.

These psychological and social characteristics are often mistaken as the person's personality whereas their true personality is being masked by the effects on the brain of being underweight.

CONCERNS ABOUT SHAPE AND WEIGHT

My confidence and feelings of self-worth are deeply rooted in the idea that I must be physically attractive, i.e., thin. When I put on weight, even 1 pound, I risk being unattractive, and I see my future as bleak and lonely. This thought fills me with despair, so I force myself to eat as little as possible.

Most people who binge are extremely concerned about their shape and weight. Indeed, these concerns may be so intense that their life becomes dominated by them; nothing else much matters. This "over-concern" is characteristic of most forms of eating disorder: indeed, many experts view it as the "core" feature as everything else seems to stem from it. The overconcern is most prominent in bulimia nervosa and anorexia nervosa and many atypical eating disorders (see Chapter 2). It is less prominent in people with binge eating disorder. Their concerns tend to have a different quality. They are better described as dissatisfaction and they are somewhat more understandable in view of these people's higher weight. Nevertheless, they can be a problem. For example, some people with binge eating disorder go to great lengths to prevent others from seeing their body, and they may also avoid seeing it themselves. Some even view their appearance with disgust and loathing.

What does overconcern about shape and weight mean? Think for a moment about how you evaluate yourself as a person. Whereas the majority of people evaluate themselves on the basis of how they are performing in a variety of areas of their life (such as the quality of their relationships, their performance at work, their athletic accomplishments, etc.), most people with an eating problem judge their self-worth largely, or even exclusively, in terms of their shape and weight and their ability to control them. This can be represented diagrammatically in the form of a pie chart in which each slice represents an area of life that is valued; the bigger the slice the more important that area is to the person concerned. Figures 10 and 11 show two such pie charts, one of a young woman with no eating problem and the other of someone with overconcern about shape and weight.

The overconcern about shape and weight seen in bulimia nervosa, anorexia nervosa, and many atypical eating disorders is of great importance in understanding these problems. It is central to their persistence—it is the "engine" that drives these problems. It accounts for the strict dieting (and therefore any binge eating), the vomiting, the misuse of laxatives and diuretics, and excessive exercising. It also accounts for a range of other phenomena that we are about to discuss. And, understandably, the overconcern is maintained by any tendency to binge eat, creating a further vicious circle (see Figure 12). Reducing the intensity of these concerns is therefore a major goal of treatment. Guidelines for doing this are provided in Part II.

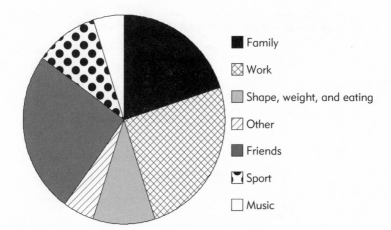

FIGURE 10. The pie chart of a young woman **without** an eating problem.

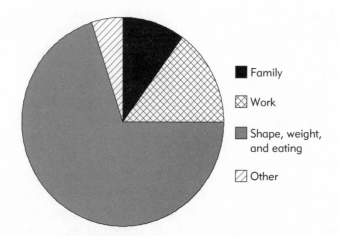

FIGURE 11. The pie chart of a young woman **with** an eating problem.

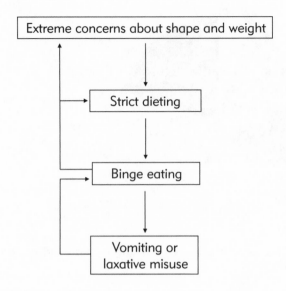

FIGURE 12. The central role of concerns about shape and weight.

Weight Checking and Weight Avoidance

> *I am obsessed with my weight. I weigh myself over and over again, sometimes up to 15 times a day. At other times I am so disgusted with my body that I don't use the scales for weeks or months at a time.*

The most direct "expression" of overconcern about weight and shape is body checking. This may involve weight checking, shape checking, or both.

Many people with binge eating problems weigh themselves at frequent intervals, sometimes many times a day. For example, over a quarter of those with bulimia nervosa weigh themselves at least once a day, compared to only one in 20 women in the community (see Figure 13). As a result many become concerned about day-to-day weight fluctuations that would otherwise pass unnoticed. This leads them to restrict their eating, whatever the number on the scales: if it is "up" or "the same," they try to diet even harder; and if it is

"down," their dieting is reinforced. Whatever the number,
they tend to conclude that

> *Short-term weight changes are not indicative of changes in body fat.*

they must continue to diet. This is yet another process that maintains binge eating problems. What is often not appreciated is that
day-to-day weight changes are not indicative of changes in body fat.
They are much more likely to be due to changes in hydration, as
explained in Chapter 5 (p. 66).

Other people with binge eating problems actively avoid knowing their weight while remaining highly concerned about it. Generally these people used to weigh themselves frequently but switched
to avoidance as they found frequent weighing too aversive. Unfortunately, avoidance of weighing is as problematic as frequent weighing
because it results in fears and assumptions about weight remaining
unchallenged.

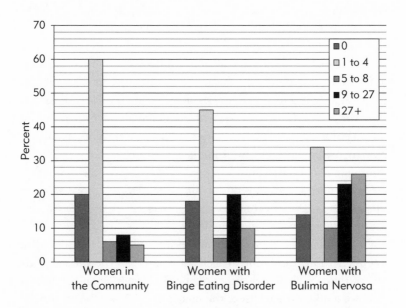

FIGURE 13. How often people weigh themselves (times per 28 days).

Shape Checking

> I am confident in many ways, yet I hate my body and can't bear to look at it. I feel bloated, wobbly, and huge all over. This drives me to binge. My boyfriend loves me. Why can't I like myself?

> Immediately I wake up I feel my hips and stomach to check that they're not covered in a layer of fat.

Shape checking is another form of body checking. Of course, everyone checks their body to some extent but many people with a binge eating problem check their body repeatedly and in ways that are unusual. They may study themselves in the mirror, measure themselves, and even take repeated photographs of themselves when unclothed. In addition, they may assess the tightness of set items of clothing or accessories (e.g., watches or rings), and they may look down at themselves when sitting to assess how much their stomach bulges out or to what extent their thighs splay. If you are male you may be concerned about your build and muscularity (or lack of it) and focus your checking on this. Such shape checking can become so "second nature" that you may not be fully aware that you are doing it; for example, when taking a shower many people are also inadvertently shape checking by feeling their bones and pinching their flesh.

Mirrors can be a particular problem. Studying yourself in the mirror is a particular form of shape checking that has the potential to provide highly credible, but misleading, information. We all believe what we see in the mirror, yet assessing oneself in a mirror is far more complex than is generally realized. To illustrate this point, consider the size of your image when you look at yourself in a full-length mirror. Is the image that you see on the surface of the mirror the same height as your true height? If not, what height is it? And what about the width of the image? To find out the answer, ask a friend to mark on the mirror surface the top and bottom of your reflection as you see it (when you are standing sufficiently far away so

> Mirrors have the potential to provide highly credible, but misleading information.

that you can see your head and feet) and then measure how far apart they are. You will find that your image on the mirror surface is about half your size in all dimensions, something that you have probably not noticed before. The fact that you have not realized that you have been looking at a very small version of yourself over all these years should help to persuade you that mirrors are complex and that a lot of mental processing goes on "behind the scenes" when you look into the mirror.

There are three points to emphasize about shape checking. First, it generally involves the studying of aspects of appearance that are disliked. This is bound to maintain body dissatisfaction. Second, when checking, what you discover depends to a large extent upon the way that you assess yourself. If people look at themselves in detail, "flaws" that would normally go unnoticed become prominent and, once noticed, they are hard to forget. Even really attractive people would find flaws if they studied themselves. And third, scrutiny is prone to magnify apparent defects. This is illustrated by a phenomenon seen among people with spider phobias. They tend to see spiders as larger than they really are.

If you look for fatness, you will find it.

This is because when looking at spiders they focus down on them and their unpleasant characteristics while not looking at the surrounding environment. As a result they get detailed information about the spider in the absence of any reference points for size. An equivalent phenomenon happens to people who study themselves in the mirror because scrutinizing aspects of one's body is prone to magnify them. If you look for fatness, you will find it: indeed, you will create it.

Comparison Making

Comparison making is a particular form of shape checking. Some people with binge eating problems do this repeatedly and usually in a way that makes them conclude that they are unattractive relative to others. This is because they make a superficial assessment of the other person while critically scrutinizing themselves. Furthermore, they tend to compare themselves with people who are thin and good-looking: they fail to notice those who are less thin and attractive.

It is also common for people with eating problems to compare themselves with photographs in magazines and on the Internet without taking into account that these images have often been manipulated. As we discuss in Part II, it is important to become street-wise in this regard (see p. 205).

Shape Avoidance

I cannot put into words how repulsed I am with my body. I cannot bear to look at it. I will have no mirrors in the house. I take showers instead of baths to avoid having to look at myself. I have not gone shopping for clothes for more than 3 years.

I can never shower with the lights on. If I do, I will see all my fat.

Shape avoidance is the counterpart to shape checking. The term refers to behavior designed to prevent the person from seeing his or her body and being aware of it. It often includes avoidance of others seeing their body too. It stems from a strong dislike of how their body looks or feels. Often people with shape avoidance used to engage in shape checking but switched to avoidance because the checking became too distressing.

Shape avoidance takes various forms: it can involve avoiding looking in the mirror, not wearing tight clothes, covering the stomach (e.g., with the arms), and not looking at photographs. It is as problematic as it is distressing and it allows concerns about shape to persist unquestioned.

When extreme, shape avoidance can profoundly interfere with day-to-day life. At the mild end it affects clothes choice, the ability to go swimming, and changing in public. At the more severe end, the person may be unable to have a sex life or any form of physical intimacy due to his or her dislike of being touched or seen. Telling these people that they look fine is rarely reassuring as most are impervious to comments of this type or they interpret them negatively.

Occasionally shape checking and avoidance coexist. When this occurs the person checks some aspects of his or her body while avoiding others, or switches from checking to avoidance and back.

Feeling Fat

Feeling fat is another product of concerns about shape and weight. Of course, feeling fat is an experience reported by many women, and some men, but its intensity and frequency is far greater among people with eating problems. It is an important phenomenon because it can be equated with actually being "fat," and when this occurs it tends to encourage dieting.

Feeling fat is ill-understood: indeed, remarkably little has been written about it. What is noteworthy is that the experience fluctuates markedly in intensity from day to day and even within a day. This is quite unlike overconcern with shape and weight, which tends to be stable, as are one's actual shape and weight.

> *Feeling fat is usually the result of mislabeling certain emotions and bodily experiences.*

Feeling fat is usually the result of mislabeling unpleasant emotions and bodily experiences. These include feeling depressed, lonely, or unloved; or feeling bloated, premenstrual, or hungover. Why this mislabeling occurs is not clear but it could be a consequence of the long-standing and profound preoccupation with thoughts about shape.

When feeling fat is frequent, intense, or distressing, it needs to be tackled in treatment. Doing so is one element of the self-help program in Part II.

OTHER PSYCHOLOGICAL AND SOCIAL PROBLEMS

My eating problem has taken over my whole life. My friendships have been upset by my violent swings in mood. I never talk to my parents since they have never understood what I am going through, yet we were so close. I have so little self-confidence. I get terribly depressed and anxious. I can't face seeing people.

My life revolves around my eating. I can no longer concentrate on my work, which has suffered as a result. My problem has caused family rows [arguments]. I no longer enjoy sharing meals with family or friends. I have become withdrawn and introspective and have lost all self-confidence and self-respect. I don't want to go out. I don't like myself anymore.

I am late for everything because eating takes so much time . . . and not just the eating part but the buying of food, getting rid of the packages, cleaning up, etc, etc.

As you will be aware if you have a binge eating problem, your quality of life suffers. You may feel depressed and demoralized. Many people are ashamed of their lack of willpower and feel guilty about their secrecy and deceit. They are highly self-critical. Some get so desperate that they attempt to take their life. Others repeatedly harm themselves, often by cutting their skin. This can be to punish themselves, to relieve tension, or both. Irritability is also common.

The feelings of depression can be severe. Generally they are secondary to the binge eating problem and when this is the case they resolve once the person regains control over his or her eating. However, in a subgroup, a true clinical depression develops. Features that suggest that this has happened include a sustained lowering of mood, loss of psychological drive, thoughts about death and dying, uncharacteristic tearfulness, and social withdrawal. If you have some or all of these features then it is important to seek professional advice as depression is serious yet eminently treatable.

Those who binge are also prone to be anxious, both as a character trait and, most especially, when in situations that activate their concerns. For example, some avoid social occasions, particularly those that involve eating. This might mean missing the wedding of a close friend or the birthday party of a parent—all of which hurt both the person with the eating problem and his or her friends or family. Events and circumstances that involve some degree of body exposure are also often avoided. These include swimming, parties, and beach vacations.

Nor is excessive drinking uncommon. This may take the form of habitual overconsumption or intermittent binge drinking. The latter is typically triggered by adverse events or moods, much like binge eating. A small minority misuses psychoactive drugs.

Two character traits are prominent among people with binge eating problems. The first is low self-esteem. Feelings of inadequacy and worthlessness are common. While they are often part of any accompanying demoralization or depression, and so improve as the eating problem resolves, they can also be the expression of a long-standing personality trait. Some people describe such feelings as stretching back into their childhoods.

The other common character trait is perfectionism. Many people who binge tend to set unduly demanding standards for themselves. Their perfectionism tends to affect most aspects of their life, but it is particularly obvious in the dietary goals that they set for themselves. The trait does, of course, have its positive side as perfectionists may perform exceptionally well at work and in other aspects of life that they value. The key issue is whether their standards are realistic. If they are, there is no problem. However, if they are not, they will experience repeated "failures" even when their performance is high by most people's standards. Failing in this way can be undermining, especially if self-esteem is low. Indeed, the combination of low self-esteem and perfectionism is not unusual among those who binge, and especially those with bulimia nervosa, anorexia nervosa, or an atypical eating disorder (see Chapter 2, p. 28), and it may well contribute to the development of the problem (see Chapter 6).

At their worst, binge eating problems affect every aspect of life. Nothing is spared. So much time and effort is taken up by the problem that little is left for anything else. Relationships with family and friends may even become unsustainable. As with the feelings of depression most interpersonal problems improve markedly, if not go away altogether, once the binge eating problem recedes. One of the most gratifying aspects of helping people overcome binge eating problems is seeing the person underneath gradually emerge as the problem goes away. The depression, tension, and irritability fade; relationships improve; and old interests return.

CHAPTER 5

Physical Aspects

As we discussed in Chapter 4, binge eating problems are associated with a diverse array of difficulties. Over time they can transform an ordinary, happy existence into a miserable one, harming not only the person with the problem but also his or her relationships with family and friends.

Binge eating problems can also affect physical health, either as a direct result of the overeating or as a consequence of any associated weight control behavior. Many of the physical effects are reversible, but some are not. Most become worse with time, so they should not be ignored. But first, some facts about body weight need to be stressed because misconceptions abound.

SOME FACTS ABOUT WEIGHT

As we discussed in Chapter 4, most people with binge eating problems are very concerned about their weight and shape. Despite this, many harbor misunderstandings about body weight. Below are some key facts about weight and weight fluctuations.

We are mainly water. About 60% of our weight (as adults) is water. So, if you weigh 160 pounds (72 kilograms), almost 100 pounds (43 kilograms) of your weight is accounted for by water.

Our weight fluctuates within the day and from day to day.

These short-term changes in weight (ranging from 1 to 3 pounds [0.5 to 1.5 kilograms]) are largely the result of changes in our level of hydration. As we are mainly water, even small changes in our hydration have a measureable effect on our weight. This phenomenon is exploited by those who participate in sports in which "making weight" is required (see Box 6). In people who vomit, or misuse laxatives or diuretics, hydration levels fluctuate considerably and as a result so does their body weight.

Short-term changes in weight do not reflect changes in body fat. As we noted above, these short-term changes are largely the result of changes in hydration. It is important to keep this is in mind when weighing yourself. In the self-help program in Part II (p. 164), there are detailed guidelines for how to interpret changes in the number on the scale.

BOX 6. Jockeys and "making weight."

In some sports participants are required to be below a particular weight at a set time in order to be allowed to compete. This is referred to as "making weight."

For jockeys, this threshold is most often 120 pounds (54 kilograms; which includes the weight of their clothes, shoes, helmet, and tack). For some jockeys, the pressure to be below a specific weight drives them to use unhealthy weight control practices on the day of races. These practices include self-induced vomiting, "sweat rooms," and other means of dehydrating themselves.

Cotugna and colleagues interviewed 20 jockeys and found that their race season BMI (see p. 26) ranged between 17.0 and 21.4, placing some in the markedly underweight BMI range. Their average weight loss on race days (days when they had to make weight) was 2.5 pounds, but some jockeys lost as much as 5 pounds. This weight loss is entirely the result of loss of water, highlighting the huge influence hydration has on body weight.

Source: Cotugna, N., Snider, O. S., & Windish, J. (2011). Nutrition assessment of horse-racing athletes. *Journal of Community Health, 36,* 261–264.

SOME FACTS ABOUT DIETING
AND WEIGHT LOSS

Many people with binge eating problems are also concerned about their diet. Some are assiduous readers of articles on food and nutrition, and many think that they are well informed. My clinical experience, however, suggests that this is often not the case. While some of my patients are knowledgeable, many others hold erroneous views acquired through years of absorbing unreliable and inconsistent sources of information. Below are some important facts about dieting and weight loss.

There is no single "healthy diet." A healthy diet is one that matches our nutritional needs and optimizes our physical health. As our nutritional needs change according to our age and other life circumstances, so does what constitutes a "healthy diet." For the majority of adults, and especially those who are middle-aged or elderly, the optimal diet is one that minimizes the risk of weight gain, heart disease, and cancer. However, a different diet is recommended for women who are pregnant and those who are breast feeding. There are also specific diets for people with health problems such as diabetes. There is no single healthy diet.

Weight-loss diets are not healthy diets. Weight-loss diets are designed to help people lose weight. They are not in and of themselves healthy, although they may help you reach a healthier weight if you are overweight (see Appendix II, p. 216).

Weight-loss diets are designed to create an energy imbalance such that your energy (calorie) intake in the form of food and drink is less than the energy needed to fuel your physical activity and to keep your body working. If this energy imbalance is sustained over time, you will lose weight.

Weight-loss diets are for people who are overweight or who have obesity. If you are not overweight, there is no reason healthwise to follow a weight-loss diet. If you have the goal of achieving an unduly low weight (a BMI below 18.5; see Part II, p. 124), then think twice. As we shall shortly discuss, being underweight adversely affects physical health and it also has major psychological and social effects.

Weight-loss diets are subject to fashion. What is "in" one year may well be "out" the next. For example, in the 1960s and 1970s carbohydrates were "bad" and were to be avoided. Then in the 1980s and 1990s dietary fat was the villain and carbohydrates were ok. In the 2000s carbohydrates were once again the enemy. And so it goes on. If there were a consistently successful way of losing weight, it would sweep aside these fashions and fads. Have a look at the U.S. National Institutes of Health website at *www.win.niddk.nih.gov/publications/ myths.htm* for a list of common myths and misunderstandings about weight loss and nutrition.

Distinguishing weight loss and weight maintenance. Weight-loss diets are not designed to be used for the long term, as they do not match our nutritional needs. Indeed, certain weight-loss diets would do you harm if you followed them for a sustained period of time.

In practice few people can follow a weight-loss diet for more than 4 or 5 months. What they then do is critical. There is a tendency to "give up" and return to their old way of eating. This results in weight regain. Instead, if they want to maintain their new lower weight, they need to move over from their weight-loss regimen to a weight maintenance one. Many weight-loss programs omit to mention this. Perhaps this is why weight regain is so common.

A healthy diet involves eating a wide variety of foods. We should also drink plenty of water. The only things we should go easy on, but not exclude, are salt, sugar, and two types of fat: saturated fat and trans fat. This is because these forms of fat increase the risk of cardiovascular disease. Saturated fats are mostly found in red meat and dairy foods whereas trans fats are found in hard margarine, fried food, and many commercially baked foods. But not all fat is of this type. What can get forgotten is that "unsaturated fat" (found in fish, seafood, nuts, and olive oil) reduces the risk of heart disease.

You may be thinking that you have heard all this before but *"How do I translate the healthy eating guidelines into real food? What should I eat?"* Until recently health educators used a "food pyramid" to explain what proportions of the various types of food make up a healthy diet. More recently the pyramid has been replaced by a plate (see *www.choosemyplate.gov*) but the overall message remains much the same.

As for how much you should eat, misunderstandings are rife. I regularly meet people who think that they ought to eat no more than 1,500 calories per day and others who think that 2,500 calories per day is about right. While I certainly would not advocate calorie counting, which can become a problem in its own right, it is important to be in the right ballpark. Table 5 lists the approximate calorie needs of adults with various lifestyles.

For up-to-date information on nutrition and healthy eating go on the web and search the various nutrition-related websites of the U.S. government and the National Institutes of Health. If you are from outside the United States, have a look at your own country's dietary recommendations as well.

Vitamins and minerals are best obtained from food. Consuming additional quantities of vitamins and the like in the form of pills or liquids is not a good idea unless you have been advised to do so by a health professional. Indeed, doing so can cause you harm (see *www. ods.od.nih.gov*).

TABLE 5. Approximate calorie needs per day (plus or minus 100 calories).

| Age (years) | | Activity level | |
	Inactive	Somewhat active	Active
		Women	
18–50	1,900	2,100	2,400
Over 50	1,600	1,800	2,100
		Men	
18–50	2,500	2,700	3,000
Over 50	2,100	2,300	2,600

You don't have to eat perfectly to be perfectly healthy. This message (adapted from one by Marcia Herrin of the Dartmouth College Eating Disorders Program) is for people who are concerned about precisely what they eat. This is not necessary. Healthy eating guidelines are exactly that: they are guidelines. They are intended to be followed in a flexible way. They should not rule your life.

PHYSICAL EFFECTS OF BINGE EATING

Effects on the Stomach

> *I stop eating when it is impossible for me to continue—when I am literally full. After a binge I feel so full that my stomach hurts and I can hardly move. I feel sick, and sometimes, when I have had a particularly bad binge, even breathing is difficult and painful.*

Binge eating has few immediate physical effects, but most binges leave the person feeling full, and in some cases the feeling is intense and painful. As Table 6 shows, people with bulimia nervosa are more likely to feel extremely full after a binge than people with binge eating disorder. This difference probably reflects their relative speed of eating.

People who eat until they are very full sometimes describe becoming breathless. This is caused by their distended stomach pressing up on the diaphragm. Very rarely, the stomach wall becomes so stretched that it is damaged or even tears. This is a serious medical emergency. If you develop abdominal pain when bingeing it is essential that you stop eating immediately. And if the pain is extreme, get help.

Binge Eating and Body Weight

The relationship between binge eating and body weight is not a simple one. In both bulimia and binge eating disorder binge eating is frequent, yet body weight is usually normal in the former condition and raised in the latter. Why is this? It is likely to be the result of the way

TABLE 6. How full people get after binge eating.

Bulimia nervosa

7%—do not feel full

7%—feel slightly uncomfortable (bloated, definite physical sense of having overeaten)

60%—feel moderately uncomfortable (distended but no pain)

26%—physically impossible to continue eating due to painful severe distension

Binge eating disorder

17%—do not feel full

32%—feel slightly uncomfortable (bloated, definite physical sense of having overeaten)

47%—feel moderately uncomfortable (distended but no pain)

4%—physically impossible to continue eating due to painful severe distension

these people eat outside their binges. Remember the eating habits of people with bulimia nervosa consist of extreme dieting punctuated by episodes of binge eating. In contrast, in binge eating disorder the binge eating occurs against the background of a general tendency to overeat. It is therefore not surprising that the majority of the former group are not overweight whereas most of the latter are.

What happens to body weight with successful treatment? In people with binge eating disorder stopping binge eating has little effect on body weight. This is because it is their overeating in general that is contributing most to their high weight. The same is true in bulimia nervosa but for a different reason. In this case it is because the better treatments for bulimia nervosa target both these people's binge eating and the accompanying dieting, with the resulting effects on weight cancelling each other out. To illustrate this finding, data from a treatment study conducted by my group in Oxford indicate that those who made a full recovery from bulimia nervosa had on average virtually no change in weight: their average weight was 137 pounds (62 kilograms) before treatment and 134 pounds (61 kilograms) 16 months later. However, it is important to note that these figures do reflect the average—some patients lost more weight than this, whereas others gained.

What about anorexia nervosa? In people with anorexia nervosa binge eating has little impact on body weight so long as the binges are relatively infrequent and "subjective" (i.e., small in size; see Chapter 2, p. 12). However, if the binges become frequent or large, they cause body weight to rise with the result that the person's eating disorder diagnosis may change from anorexia nervosa to bulimia nervosa (again, see Chapter 2).

PHYSICAL EFFECTS OF DIETING

Besides having the psychological effects described in Chapter 4, dieting can have adverse physical effects. For example, it has been suggested that repeated cycles of weight loss and regain (weight cycling)—sometimes called "yo-yo dieting"—alter body composition and metabolism in ways that make subsequent attempts to lose weight more difficult.

Dieting may also affect menstruation as regular menstruation requires a certain minimum amount of body fat. It is for this reason almost all women with anorexia nervosa do not menstruate (see Box 7). Even when the amount of body fat is adequate, dieting, irregular eating, and intense exercising all have an influence on menstruation, although the mechanisms responsible are unclear. Menstrual disturbance is seen in up to half of those with bulimia nervosa and in about one in four women with binge eating disorder.

PHYSICAL EFFECTS
OF SELF-INDUCED VOMITING

As we discussed in Chapter 4, self-induced vomiting is common in bulimia nervosa. It also occurs in anorexia nervosa, particularly

---

BOX 7. Could mannequins menstruate?

Investigators from Helsinki, Finland, measured the height and other dimensions of mannequins from the 1920s on. They calculated their percentage of body fat as if they had been real women. Before the 1950s the amount of body fat was mostly in the normal range. Thereafter, it was considerably less. They concluded that a woman with the shape of a modern mannequin would be unlikely to menstruate.

Source: Rintala, M., & Mustajoki, P. (1992). Could mannequins menstruate? *British Medical Journal, 305,* 1575–1576.

---

among those who binge, and it is also common among those with atypical eating disorders.

Not surprisingly, repeated self-induced vomiting has a number of adverse physical effects. These are seen most often among those who vomit frequently and have done so for some time. As explained here, some of these effects are potentially serious.

Damage to the Teeth. Repeated vomiting over a long period of time damages the teeth; it gradually erodes the dental enamel mainly on the inner surface of the front teeth. Dental fillings are not affected so they become prominent relative to the surface of the enamel. Dentists can readily identify this pattern of erosion and may therefore deduce its cause. The erosion is irreversible but not progressive—in other words, it stops once the vomiting stops. The practice of rinsing the mouth with water after vomiting is thought to accelerate the dental erosion rather than retard it.

Swelling of the Salivary Glands. Surrounding the mouth are glands that produce saliva. In some people who induce vomiting these glands gradually swell. The swelling is painless, but it may increase the production of saliva. Often it is the parotid gland (the gland commonly affected in mumps) that swells most, giving the person's face a somewhat rounded, chubby appearance. People with parotid swelling tend to see their face as "fat" and may assume that the rest of their body looks the same way. Naturally this increases their concern about shape and weight, thereby perpetuating the eating problem. The swelling of the salivary glands is reversible and gradually goes away as eating habits improve.

Damage to the Throat. As described in Chapter 4, most people induce vomiting by mechanically stimulating the gag reflex. This can be a difficult and long process requiring some force. Superficial injuries to the back of the throat can result, and these may get infected. Complaints of recurrent sore throats and hoarseness are therefore not uncommon.

Damage to the Esophagus. Very rarely, violent vomiting tears the wall of the esophagus, the tube that leads from the mouth to the stomach. There is a remote risk of rupture of the esophagus. This is a medical emergency. If there is a significant amount of fresh blood in your vomit you must seek medical advice.

Damage to the Hands. One other mechanical effect of self-induced vomiting is seen in some people who use their fingers to stimulate the gag reflex. It is damage to the skin over the knuckles of the hand. Initially abrasions appear on the hand due to it rubbing against the teeth, and eventually scars form. This is a highly characteristic abnormality known in medical textbooks as "Russell's sign" because it was first described by Gerald Russell in his classic paper on bulimia nervosa.

Fluid and Electrolyte Imbalance. The physiological effects of frequent vomiting can be serious, and especially so among those who attempt to "wash out" their stomach by repeatedly drinking and vomiting until there is no sign of food in what they are bringing up. Repeated vomiting affects hydration, as I discussed earlier (p. 67), and electrolyte levels too (sodium, potassium, etc.). The electrolyte disturbance of most concern is hypokalemia (low potassium) since it can result in potentially dangerous heart beat irregularities. If your heart beat is irregular you should seek the advice of a physician.

The symptoms of fluid or electrolyte disturbance include

extreme thirst, dizziness, swelling of the legs and arms, weakness and lethargy, muscle twitches and spasms, and even epileptic seizures. Although up to half of those with bulimia nervosa have fluid and electrolyte abnormalities of some sort, most have none of these symptoms, and the disturbance is mild. It is also important to note that all these symptoms can have other causes so their presence is not necessarily indicative of an underlying fluid or electrolyte abnormality.

Electrolyte disturbance is reversible; it promptly goes away once vomiting stops. Rarely does it require treatment in its own right, and any treatment should be supervised by a physician. You should never try to treat it yourself.

A small number of people induce vomiting chemically. For example, they may drink salt water to make themselves sick. This is particularly inadvisable since it is another cause of electrolyte disturbance. Others take the over-the-counter drug Ipecac (ipecacuanha) to induce vomiting, a dangerous practice because several toxic effects can result from its use.

PHYSICAL EFFECTS OF LAXATIVE MISUSE

As explained in Chapter 4, people who binge may take laxatives to influence their shape and weight, though the practice is less common than self-induced vomiting. It is pursued mainly by people with bulimia nervosa or anorexia nervosa. Some people take very large quantities, as many as 50 to a 100 at a time.

Laxatives have little effect on calorie absorption.

Regardless of the amount taken, laxatives have little effect on calorie absorption. They act on the lower part of the intestine, whereas calories are absorbed higher up. What they do produce is watery diarrhea and a temporary fall in weight due to the loss of water. (Recall that about 60% of our weight is accounted for by water.) However, the weight loss is short-lived because the person regains the lost weight almost immediately as his or her body rehydrates. Nevertheless, people with bulimia nervosa find the weight loss rewarding, believing erroneously that it is evidence of an effect on calorie absorption.

Laxative misuse, much like self-induced vomiting, produces a variety of fluid and electrolyte abnormalities with symptoms of the type just described. Individuals who both vomit and misuse laxatives are at particular risk. Some laxatives, when taken in high doses over long periods, result in permanent damage to the intestine. Generally, however, the adverse physical effects are reversible.

People who have taken laxatives on a regular basis for some time may retain fluid (water) for a week or so if they stop abruptly. Doing so results in temporary weight gain which can be distressing, and it may lead them to resume laxative taking. It is important that people realize that the weight gain is due to water retention, not fat, and that it will go away within a week or so at the most.

PHYSICAL EFFECTS OF DIURETIC MISUSE

Some people take diuretics (water tablets), usually over-the-counter preparations, in an attempt to change their shape and weight. This is a fruitless exercise since diuretics have no effect on calorie absorption. Like laxatives, they cause fluid loss, in this case through the production of excess urine, and thus they have a short-lived effect on body weight. When taken in large quantities, they can produce fluid and electrolyte disturbance which, as previously mentioned, can be dangerous. Again, this is reversible. As with laxatives, those who stop taking diuretics after having used them for some time may experience temporary fluid retention.

PHYSICAL EFFECTS OF EXCESSIVE EXERCISE

As we noted in Chapter 4, some people with binge eating problems exercise a lot, in large part to influence their shape or weight. This does not usually have adverse physical effects unless it is contributing to them having an unduly low body weight (see below) or it results in "overuse injuries." Certain types of exercise (e.g., horse riding) can be particularly risky in anorexia nervosa where there is a heightened risk of bone fractures.

PHYSICAL EFFECTS OF BEING UNDERWEIGHT

Being underweight has many diverse effects on physical health. Their nature depends upon the extent and form of the dietary deprivation.

Brain. Those who are underweight often overlook the fact that they are adversely affecting their brain, both its structure and its functioning. Starting with structure, it has been found in anorexia nervosa that the brain's grey matter and white matter are both significantly reduced in size. Dieting does not spare the brain—it too is affected. As regards brain function, the brain requires a considerable amount of energy (i.e., calories) to operate properly, something that is in short supply among those who are undereating.

Given these effects of undereating, it is hardly surprising that cognitive and emotional deficits are common in those with anorexia nervosa, and in others who undereat (as we discussed in Chapter 4), abnormalities that are reversed by weight restoration.

Circulation. There are profound effects on the heart and circulation. Heart muscle is lost and the heart is weaker as a result. Blood pressure drops and the heart rate (pulse) declines. There is heightened risk of serious heart beat irregularities (arrhythmias), especially if there are accompanying disturbances in fluid and electrolytes. If your heart beat is irregular or unusually slow (less than 50 beats per minute), you should seek the advice of a physician.

Hormones. Likewise there are profound effects on hormonal function with nonessential processes ceasing. As a result sex hormone production declines markedly and women become infertile (see later in this chapter). There is a loss of appetite for sex and sexual responsiveness declines.

Bones. There is deterioration in bone strength. This is in part due to the hormonal changes, in part due to the decrease in the weight that the bones have to carry, and in part a direct dietary effect. The result is an increased risk of osteoporosis and fractures.

Digestive System. There may be a persistent sense of hunger although this is far from invariable. The sense of taste may be impaired, with the result that some people use large quantities of condiments and spices to give flavor to their food. The gut slows down, presumably so that food absorption is maximized. Thus, food in the stomach takes much longer than normal to move into the small intestine. This may also account in part for why people who are underweight have a heightened sensation of fullness even after eating relatively little.

Muscles. These waste, and weakness can result. This is most obvious when walking up stairs or trying to stand up from a sitting or squatting position.

Skin and Hair. The effects vary. A downy hair (called lanugo) may start to grow on the body, especially on the face, abdomen, back, and arms. There may also be hair loss from the scalp. Often the skin becomes dry and it can develop an orange tinge.

Temperature Regulation. The main change is a decrease in body temperature. Some people feel profoundly cold.

Sleep. Sleep is also impaired. It is less refreshing, and there is a tendency to wake early.

EFFECTS ON FERTILITY AND PREGNANCY

I worry about my eating problem affecting my relationship with my baby and my ability to cope. I hope to have three children, but I don't like the idea of getting pregnant again. Maybe next time I won't still be bulimic.

I had done really well with my eating. I had stopped vomiting and taking laxatives the moment I found out I was pregnant. I had also stopped binge eating. And I was trying really hard to eat only healthy foods. And then I was examined by my doctor and, when he was feeling my tummy, he looked up at me and said, "I am sorry I am taking so long, but I can't tell which is the baby and which is you." I know he was just joking, but it really upset me. I went home and cried. I ate nothing at all for the next few days, and when, with my husband's help, I did start eating again, I found that I could no longer resist vomiting afterwards.

I try to control my eating but find it difficult. After making myself vomit I feel extremely guilty as I would never forgive myself if any harm came to my baby—but I am pleased that I have stopped taking laxatives.

Binge eating problems are associated with impaired fertility (see Box 8), but the reasons for this are not clear. Certainly, dieting, weight loss, and a low body weight all affect fertility, but it is not known whether binge eating has an effect too. What is important to stress is that these effects are generally reversible so long as the eating problem is overcome.

Similarly, little is known about the effects of binge eating problems on pregnancy. Most of the research has looked at bulimia nervosa. The findings suggest that the binge eating generally improves once the woman knows that she is pregnant. The desire not to harm the fetus is strong, and for some it is sufficiently powerful to prevent them from binge eating throughout pregnancy. Self-induced vomiting also tends to decline in frequency and most people stop misusing laxatives. Interestingly, dietary cravings occur, just as in other people's pregnancies. These cravings can lead to the consumption of foods that would otherwise be avoided (such as ice cream) and, as a result, they can trigger binges.

BOX 8. The "Dutch Hunger Winter."

Before babies are born their subsequent development is determined to an extent by the environment in the womb. This prepares them for the circumstances that they are likely to face when born. Some of the changes cannot be reversed and may have a lifelong impact. If, for example, the developing fetus does not receive adequate nutrition, aspects of its metabolism and physiology may alter to prepare it for an environment in which food is scarce. For example, the baby may become particularly good at laying down fat. But if circumstances subsequently alter or, for some reason, the inadequate supply of nutrients was not the result of food shortage, the developmental changes may be detrimental to long-term health.

The "Dutch Hunger Winter" was a famine that took place in the Netherlands during the Second World War when, as a reprisal for Dutch resistance, fuel and food transport to the country was banned. At the height of the famine rations fell to between 400 and 800 calories per person per day. Studies of the Dutch Hunger Winter show that, despite being born with a normal weight, women exposed to the famine during the early stages of their fetal life were more likely to have obesity at age 50 years than those who were exposed to the famine later in fetal life or not at all. Early exposure to the famine was also associated with a threefold increase in the risk of having coronary heart disease by age 50 years in both men and women.

Sources: Painter, R. C., Roseboom, T. J., & Bleker, O. P. (2005). Prenatal exposure to the Dutch famine and disease in later life: An overview. *Reproductive Toxicology, 20,* 345–352.

Ravelli, A. C., van der Meulen, J. H. P., Osmond, C., Barker, D. J. P., & Bleker, O. P. (1999). Obesity at the age of 50 in men and women exposed to famine prenatally. *American Journal of Clinical Nutrition, 70,* 811–816.

Roseboom, T. J., van der Meulen, J. H. P., Osmond, C., et al. (2000). Coronary heart disease after prenatal exposure to the Dutch famine, 1944–45. *Heart, 84,* 595–598.

Although I really wanted to control my eating, it was very difficult as my body seemed to take over in certain ways. I had cravings for foods that I would never normally eat. I found that I had to submit to them from time to time, which made me feel extremely guilty.

From midpregnancy onward many women with binge eating problems experience some degree of reprieve from their concerns about their appearance and weight. They feel that they are no longer accountable for them; changes in their appearance and weight are inevitable. As a result, some abandon controlling their food intake and overeat instead. This puts them at risk of excessive weight gain which increases the risk of pregnancy complications. It also means that there will be more weight to lose following the birth.

As my pregnancy progressed, I still tried to control what I ate, calorie counting all the time and attempting to keep under 1,500 calories a day. I also exercised every day. I still had regular binges although deep down I didn't want to cause any harm to my baby. I even had a binge the day that my labor pains began.

On the other hand, a minority remain just as concerned about their appearance and weight, if not more so. The prospect of any change in shape and weight terrifies them, and they fight it. They diet, and some exercise heavily, sometimes as a substitute for vomiting or taking laxatives. As a result, they gain little or no weight, and at birth their babies may be underweight. This has the potential to have adverse long-term consequences for the child (see Box 8).

Following Childbirth

It is now 3 months since I gave birth. I've never felt so exhausted. I try to go for a run three to four times a week and I do lots of stomach exercises. I'd like to lose 15 pounds to get back into my prepregnant clothes. So far, my attempts at dieting have failed. My eating was very controlled when I first came home, but gradually the binges have returned and they are once again part of my daily life.

Following childbirth everything changes. Many find that the improvement in the binge eating problem was temporary and that it returns with a vengeance. This is not surprising as some are determined to get back to their original weight as quickly as possible and therefore resume strict dieting almost immediately. This is their downfall since, as discussed earlier, strict dieting makes people prone to binge and adhering to a diet is particularly difficult at this stressful time. Many will be breastfeeding and so subject to increased physiological pressures to eat; some will be depressed, which makes dieting difficult; and almost all will find their old routines disrupted.

CHAPTER 6

What Causes Binge Eating Problems?

I began binge eating when I was about 17. I was lonely, shy, and lacking in self-esteem. Every binge made me feel worse, made me hate myself more. I punished myself with more and more food. Within months I was binge eating as a matter of course and I gained weight rapidly. I loathed myself and continued with ordinary life only by pretending to be "normal."

Circumstances improved, and I binged less. However, my eating habits remained atrocious. Food was always on my mind. I never admitted my problems to anyone. And I lied to myself—denying what I had eaten or that I had eaten at all. Now, looking back on it all, I think of the years (almost 16) wasted, thinking about food and how fat I am. So many years spent depressed and hating myself.

Stories like this one raise an obvious two-part question: Why did this binge eating problem develop, and why did it persist for so long? Unfortunately, there is no simple, or complete, answer. Our understanding of the cause of binge eating problems is still limited.

WHY THE QUESTION IS SO DIFFICULT TO ANSWER

Many Processes Are Involved

Psychological, social, and physical processes all seem to play a part in causing binge eating problems. Chapter 3 mentioned, for example, that bulimia nervosa seems to have emerged only recently (p. 34). This suggests that environmental processes play a role and that these are likely to be social in nature. However, because not everyone develops a binge eating problem, despite being subject to similar social conditions, additional processes must also be involved. We have also seen that some psychological processes appear to be relevant such as the low self-esteem and perfectionism mentioned in Chapter 4 (p. 65). And, as this chapter shows, genetically determined processes also appear to make a contribution, which means that physical processes play a role too.

Binge Eating Problems Vary in How They Start

The research that has been done on the development of binge eating problems suggests that there is more than one route to these problems.

People with bulimia nervosa generally report that their eating problem started when they began dieting during their teenage years. This may have been provoked by a real or perceived weight problem or by a need to feel "in control" in the context of difficulties in their life. In some cases incidental weight loss (perhaps due to illness) was the trigger. Whatever the precipitant, the result is weight loss, which can be so marked that the person develops anorexia nervosa. Then, after a variable length of time, control over eating breaks down, binge eating develops, and body weight increases to near its original level.

A very different pathway is described by many people with binge eating disorder. They report a long-standing tendency to overeat, particularly when feeling unhappy or stressed. This tendency eventually becomes so marked that they develop frank episodes of binge eating. However, the binge eating tends to be phasic, that is, there are extended periods free from binge eating. This is most unlike bulimia nervosa.

To complicate matters further, some people report a mixture of these pathways especially if they have a mixed eating disorder (see Chapter 2, p. 31).

Binge Eating Problems Vary in Their Course

Binge eating problems vary in their course over time. For some, the binge eating problem is short lived and does not recur. For others, recurrences and relapses are common. For others still, once the problem begins it lasts for years. This suggests that additional processes, often separate from those that were responsible for the binge eating at the outset, come into play to keep the problem going.

What processes govern whether a binge eating problem persists or remits is not clear. In Chapter 4 we discussed the contributions of strict dieting, all-or-nothing thinking, and concerns about shape and weight. As we will see in this chapter, difficulties with relationships also seem relevant, as do certain events and circumstances.

A CRUCIAL DISTINCTION

When thinking about the cause of enduring difficulties, such as binge eating problems, it is important to distinguish the processes that are likely to have caused the problem to start in the first place from those that lead it to persist. So the question of cause has two parts:

1. Why do binge eating problems develop?
2. Why do they persist?

Two phases therefore need to be distinguished: the development phase (before the onset of the problem) and the maintenance phase (after its onset).

Making this distinction not only helps us understand the role of all possible causes but it also has significant practical implications. If the goal is the prevention of binge eating problems, the task is to identify those processes that exert their influence before onset—during the development phase—and try to stop them from operating. In contrast, if successful treatment is the goal, the task is to identify the processes that are keeping the problem going.

PROCESSES THAT CONTRIBUTE TO THE
DEVELOPMENT OF BINGE EATING PROBLEMS

Social Processes

As Chapter 3 discussed, bulimia nervosa appears to have emerged in the 1970s and 1980s in those parts of the world where anorexia nervosa was already encountered, mainly North America, northern Europe, Australia, and New Zealand. Because these are countries where it is fashionable for women to be slim, and where dieting among young women is common, social processes that encourage dieting may have contributed to the emergence of the disorder. Key among these is the shape of fashion models. Bulimia nervosa emerged when being *extremely thin*, like the English model Twiggy, became fashionable. But it is not unlikely that in different cultures different processes may contribute to the problem. Nor is the situation static as research from Fiji shows (see Box 9).

Recently, there has been a move to counter the impact of underweight fashion models. In 2006 Spain banned models with a BMI below 18.0 and in the same year Italy required the fashion industry to provide medical proof that their models did not have an eating disorder. In 2012 Israel banned models from advertisements or fashion shows if their BMI was below 18.5; and a similar line was taken by the fashion magazine *Vogue*. Unfortunately, there are forces working in the opposite direction. For example, some activities encourage unhealthy weight control practices and may as a result promote eating problems. This is particularly true of those in which a certain (low) weight is required at a specific time (e.g., horse racing—see Chapter 5, Box 6, p. 67) or where appearance is crucial, as in ballet (see Box 10).

Gender

In Chapter 3 we discussed the fact that all the eating disorders other than binge eating disorder are much more common among women than men. This pattern of women being disproportionately affected is mirrored across all cultures and ethnic groups. Why should women be

---

BOX 9. Culture change: lessons from Fiji.

Until the 1990s the Fijian islands were largely isolated from external social influences. They maintained a strong traditional culture that valued appetite and a healthy body size. Indeed, a robust body was valued. But perhaps the most protective feature of traditional Fijian culture was that people generally accepted their bodies.

In 1995, television broadcasting Western channels reached Fiji and an "explosion" of eating problems followed. One explanation is that the spread of Western culture led girls in particular to place new emphasis on their bodies, causing them the same dissatisfaction that is found in girls in the West. However, it has been argued that this explanation is too simple and that the particular nature of the clash between Western culture and Fijian values should also be considered. The islands were undergoing a major social transition at the time and this created concerns about achievement and social position. Interviews with Fijian schoolgirls suggest that many associated the slimness of Western actresses with power and success. Simultaneously, concerns about the health risks associated with obesity were promoting an emphasis on personal responsibility for body shape and weight. Therefore it seems likely that a variety of complex interacting processes were involved.

Source: Becker, A. E. (2004). Television, disordered eating and young women in Fiji: Negotiating body image and identity during rapid social change. *Culture, Medicine and Psychiatry, 28*, 533–559.

---

at greater risk? One major reason is likely to be the fact that dieting is so much more common among women than men and, as we will discuss, dieting greatly increases the risk of developing eating problems.

This raises another question: Why do women tend to diet more than men? Two answers come to mind. First, the social pressures to be slim are focused largely on women. And second, women are more prone to base their self-worth on their appearance. Both of these observations raise important wider issues concerning differences between male and female development and the competing and conflicting roles of women in Western societies.

Ethnic Group and Social Class

When patients in treatment are considered, bulimia nervosa and anorexia nervosa seem to be largely confined to Caucasian women, but patient samples are biased with respect to ethnicity. The findings of community-based studies suggest that binge eating problems are

---

BOX 10. Body image and classical ballet.

In the world of ballet the "Balanchine body," which consists of a thin frame, long legs, a long neck, and a short torso, represents the ideal. This aesthetic is attributed to George Balanchine who was a dancer, teacher, and celebrated choreographer. It is reported that Balanchine told his dancers that he "must see the bones" and they should "eat nothing." Whether or not this is true, there continues to be pressure on ballerinas to achieve this body type. The success of their careers depends upon it.

A recent review of *The Nutcracker* in *The New York Times* commented that one of the dancers looked as if she had "eaten one sugar plum too many." The "Nutrition Policy" of The Royal Ballet School in London acknowledges the risk of eating problems among aspiring ballet dancers. But while the school aims to promote healthy attitudes concerning weight, eating and body image, it concedes that the pressure to be thin cannot be completely removed.

The average BMI of a ballerina is somewhere around 18.5, meaning that many are close to being clinically underweight, and a substantial number have BMIs within the anorexia nervosa range (44.3% in one study). Studies also show that many ballet dancers want to lose further weight, do not menstruate, and experience a level of body dissatisfaction somewhere between that of girls in the general population and those diagnosed with anorexia nervosa.

Sources: Ringham, R., Klump, K., Kaye, W., Stone, D., Libman, S., Stowe, S., & Marcus, M. (2006). Eating disorder symptomatology among ballet dancers. *International Journal of Eating Disorders, 39*, 503–508.

Bettle, N., Bettle, O., Neumärker, U., & Neumärker, K.- J. (1998). Adolescent ballet school students: Their quest for body weight change. *Psychopathology, 31*, 153–159.

much more evenly dispersed. As far as social class is concerned, there is similarly evidence of a social class skew, with patients with bulimia nervosa and anorexia nervosa being disproportionally more common among those with a middle- or upper-class background. But this may be due to a bias in treatment-seeking with people from middle- and upper-class backgrounds being more likely to enter treatment.

Age, Adolescence, and Puberty

There is strong evidence that binge eating problems usually develop during teenage years or in early adulthood. This age of onset can probably be attributed to the fact that dieting among women is particularly common at this age. The dieting, in turn, is likely to be the result of two forces. First, as already mentioned, women are more prone than men to judge their self-worth in terms of their appearance, and this is particularly true in this age group. Second, at puberty many young women begin to develop a body shape that deviates from that considered fashionable.

This is not the same for men. Although men are under pressure to look a certain way, male puberty creates an appearance that society desires. As boys go through puberty their musculature and height increase and their shoulders become broader.

Adolescence itself may also be relevant. As we all know, this stage in life presents major developmental challenges: changing appearance, fluctuations in mood, and changes in social expectations and roles. Teenagers who have the personality traits thought to put people at risk of developing binge eating problems—perfectionism and low self-esteem—are more prone to experience a sense of loss of control at this time. Some find that dieting helps restore their sense of being in control and, as a behavior considered socially desirable by their peers, it also gives them a sense of achievement. For them, dieting may be more about self-control than anything else.

The timing of pubertal changes in relation to one's peers may also be important. It is thought that early development in girls may heighten their risk of emotional difficulties because it increases the probability that they will have to confront new problems and expectations before they are ready to do so. Additionally, the changes in shape may be particularly difficult to cope with if they occur prior to the rest of their peer group.

Certain age-dependent life changes are also relevant. A particularly important one is leaving home to go away to college. It is not at all uncommon for eating problems to develop or worsen at this time. It is easy to see why this occurs. Not only is the home-to-college transition a stressful one, but for some teenagers it is the first time that they have had full control over what and when they eat. As a result some go through a phase of unchecked undereating while others overeat and gain substantial amounts of weight.

Obesity

Research findings indicate that there is a raised rate of childhood and parental obesity among people who develop bulimia nervosa, and the same appears to be true of those with binge eating disorder. Naturally any tendency to be overweight during the childhood or teenage years is likely to magnify concerns about body shape and weight, and thereby encourage dieting. In addition, having a family member with a significant weight problem may sensitize people to "fatness" and dieting, making them strive to avoid it by restricting their eating.

Eating Problems and Disorders within the Family

It is well established that eating disorders run in families. The close relatives of a person with an eating disorder have an increased risk of developing one themselves. This could be due to genetic factors, and the research findings do indeed suggest that there is a significant genetic contribution. This said, what is inherited is not known. There are many possibilities, including the tendency to be a particular weight, biological or psychological responses to dieting, and certain personality traits. Nor is it clear which specific genes are likely to be involved. It is not unlikely that "epigenetic" processes contribute; for example, dieting may alter gene expression.

The fact that eating disorders run in families does not necessar-

ily indicate that inherited factors are wholly or even partly responsible. Aggregation within families could be due to environmental
influences. A number of studies have been done concerning the eating habits and attitudes of the family members of those with eating
problems. To date these studies have mainly focused on the relatives
of patients with anorexia nervosa, and their findings have varied
greatly. Some have found high rates of unusual eating attitudes and
behavior; others have not.

In clinical practice accounts of apparent contagion are not
uncommon. An example is mothers putting pressure on their daughters to join them on a diet (see Box 11).

Other Psychiatric Disorders within the Family

The possibility that other psychiatric disorders in the family might
contribute to eating disorders has also been studied. Most of this work
has focused on people with anorexia nervosa or bulimia nervosa.

BOX 11. Mothers, daughters, and disturbed eating.

Two groups of mothers and daughters were identified on the basis of
the daughters' scores on a widely used measure of disturbed eating.
There was a high-scoring group and, for comparison purposes, a low-
scoring group. The average age of the daughters was 16 years and the
mothers was 43 years.

The mothers of the daughters with disturbed eating differed from
the comparison mothers in the following noteworthy ways:

1. They had more disturbed eating habits.
2. They thought that their daughters should lose more weight.
3. They were more critical of their daughters' appearance.

These findings suggest that the transmission of eating disorders within
families may be, at least in part, due to contagion.

Source: Pike, K. M., & Rodin, J. (1991). Mothers, daughters, and disordered eating. *Journal of Abnormal Psychology, 100,* 198–204.

The psychiatric disorder that has been most widely studied is clinical depression. The findings suggest that the presence of depression within a family increases the risk that daughters will develop an eating problem. We do not know what mechanism might be responsible for this association. On the one hand, there could be a common underlying physiological abnormality, such as a defect in the regulation of serotonin in the brain, a chemical thought to be involved in both depression and the control of food intake. On the other hand, it could be the environmental influence on the child of being brought up by a depressed parent.

The other disorder to have been studied is psychoactive substance abuse (i.e., alcohol or drug abuse). The findings are discussed in Chapter 7.

Events and Disorders during Childhood

Clinicians who work with those with binge eating problems cannot fail to notice how common it is for traumatic events to have occurred during their patients' childhoods. Deaths, separations, parental disharmony, physical illnesses, teasing, sexual and physical abuse, and bullying all seem to occur with disturbing frequency. However, research indicates that such events occur no more often among these patients than among those with other psychiatric disorders, suggesting that they increase the risk of developing a psychiatric disorder, but not necessarily an eating disorder.

It has also been found that there is an increased rate of psychiatric problems before the onset of the eating problem. Anxiety problems are particularly common and a small subgroup has a history of childhood depression.

Personality Characteristics

As I mentioned in Chapter 4, certain personality traits seem to be common among those who develop binge eating problems. Most of the research on this topic has focused on people with bulimia nervosa or anorexia nervosa. Its relevance to binge eating disorder is uncertain.

Those who develop bulimia nervosa or anorexia nervosa are unusually compliant and conscientious as children. They are often somewhat shy and solitary, and they may have had difficulty mixing with other children. In addition, they tend to be competitive and achievement-oriented. They set themselves high standards and work hard to meet them. These traits seem to be the precursors of the low self-esteem and perfectionism seen in many people with anorexia nervosa or bulimia nervosa.

Exploratory psychotherapy often confirms these findings. Michael Strober from UCLA, a leading expert on personality and eating disorders, has stated that a detailed investigation of these patients' inner worlds reveals "the omnipresent fear of seeming weak, inadequate and average; the inability to take pleasure in leisure; a reluctance to confront risks and novelty, to engage in uninhibited spontaneous action, or to assert feelings; and the experiencing of impulses and desires as wasteful distractions to achieving higher moral objectives." Michael Strober argues that personality character-istics of this type result in these people being "hopelessly ill prepared" for the developmental demands of adolescence.

The personality characteristics of those who develop binge eat-ing disorder have not been characterized so thoroughly. Problems with assertiveness and low self-esteem seem to be especially common, whereas perfectionism seems more restricted to those who develop anorexia nervosa, bulimia nervosa, or an atypical eating disorder.

Dieting

In Chapter 4 we discussed the link between binge eating and strict dieting and the fact that both perpetuate each other (p. 42). How-ever, dieting also increases the risk of developing a binge eating prob-lem in the first place; indeed, it is a well-substantiated risk factor for anorexia nervosa and bulimia nervosa. It seems less relevant to binge eating disorder. Still, we know that the majority of those who diet do not develop eating problems. Therefore, other factors of the type already mentioned must somehow interact with dieting in the etio-logical process. Also, it may be that only certain forms of dieting are prone to put people at risk.

The Bottom Line: There Is No Single Cause

To conclude, there is no single cause of binge eating problems. There are a variety of risk factors and a variety of modes of onset. If you have a binge eating problem a multitude of factors are likely to have contributed to its development. However, as we shall now see, rather fewer processes are likely to be causing it to persist.

PROCESSES THAT PERPETUATE BINGE EATING PROBLEMS

The research on how binge eating problems change over time and what factors influence their course suggests that a limited number of interacting processes are involved. These are illustrated in Figure 14 and are discussed in turn.

Ongoing Dieting

In Chapter 4 we considered the various ways in which dieting makes people prone to binge. If the dieting is "extreme" (i.e., if the dieter exercises such restraint that he or she eats very little), strong physiological pressures will come to bear. And if the dieting is "strict" (the dieter sets highly specific dietary goals and holds an all-or-nothing attitude toward them), he or she will tend to swing between dieting and binge eating, with each promoting the other. Through these mechanisms, ongoing dieting seems to maintain many binge eating problems. It is for this reason that many treatments focus on eliminating or moderating dieting. This especially applies to treatments for anorexia nervosa, bulimia nervosa, and the atypical eating disorders. It is less relevant to binge eating disorder as in most cases there is little or no dieting.

Various factors encourage dieting, the main ones being the need to feel in "control" mentioned earlier and the influence of concerns about appearance and weight. Again, as discussed earlier, these concerns are reinforced by Western society's preference for a slim body shape. People who have been overweight in the past may be particu-

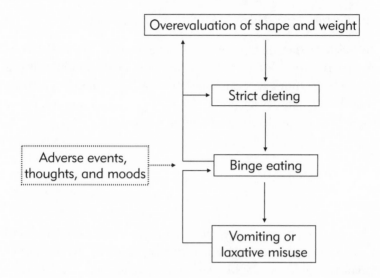

FIGURE 14. The vicious cycles that maintain binge eating.

larly likely to diet for fear of regaining their lost weight, and their efforts may be encouraged by friends and relatives.

Vomiting and the Misuse of Laxatives

Both of these methods of weight control encourage binge eating because belief in their effectiveness neutralizes a major deterrent against binge eating, namely, the fear of weight gain. This faith is unfounded, however, as we discussed in Chapter 4.

Adverse Moods and Thoughts

Mood and eating are linked in everyone, not just in those with eating problems. But binge eating has a particularly complex and circular relationship with mood. People who binge find that their binge eating helps them cope with adverse moods and thoughts because it is both distracting and calming. In this way some can come to rely on binge eating to cope with such thoughts and feelings, while being unaware of the link.

Relationships, Events, and Circumstances

A variety of events and circumstances also influence the course of binge eating problems. Personal relationships are particularly important in this regard. For example, establishing a close and accepting relationship with a partner may improve self-esteem, decrease concerns about shape and weight, and remove some sources of stress, thereby promoting recovery. The breakdown of a relationship can have the opposite effect.

Desire to Change

The processes just discussed do not constitute an exhaustive list. In fact our discussion of the processes contributing to the persistence of binge eating problems omitted one key factor, namely, the desire to change. Some people seem to have little desire to change. They accept their binge eating problem and adjust their life around it. In such cases the problem tends to persist, often year in, year out. Others decide to change, to make a fresh start and, interestingly, having made the decision, some are able to overcome the problem without outside help. Others, however, cannot.

What stimulates people to decide to change—to make a fresh start—has not been studied, but it should be. One of my hopes is that reading this book might provide some readers with just such a stimulus.

CHAPTER 7

Binge Eating and Addiction

One question we did not address in Chapter 6 is whether binge eating is an addiction. If you have ever experienced the sense of loss of control and urge to eat associated with binge eating, this question might well have crossed your mind. Or you might have read about binge eating being an addiction. Widely used terms such as *compulsive overeating* and *food addiction* certainly suggest that this is the case. In fact this view has such a strong following in the United States that it is the basis for certain prominent treatment programs.

For these reasons, it is important to consider whether binge eating should be viewed as a form of addiction. If it is not, then treatment programs based on this premise may well not be appropriate. This chapter focuses on three main questions:

1. Is it right to view binge eating as an addiction?
2. Is there any relationship between the known addictions, such as alcohol and drug abuse, and binge eating?
3. Are there implications of this view for the treatment of binge eating problems?

THE THEORY OF BINGE EATING
AS AN ADDICTION

OA believes that compulsive overeating is a threefold disease: physical, emotional and spiritual. We regard it as an addiction which, like alcoholism and drug abuse, can be arrested but not cured.

—*Overeaters Anonymous leaflet*

According to the theory that binge eating is a form of addiction—the so-called "addiction model" of binge eating—binge eating is the result of an underlying physiological process equivalent to that responsible for alcoholism. People who binge are biologically vulnerable to certain foods (typically sugar and starches) and as a result become "addicted" to them. These foods are "toxic" to these people who, as a result, are unable to control their intake so their consumption progressively rises. Since this vulnerability is biologically based, they can never be cured of the problem (or "illness"): rather, they have to learn to accept it and adjust their lives accordingly.

The concept of addiction has been debased.

Is the addiction model valid? As Terence Wilson of Rutgers University has stressed, nowadays "the concept of addiction has been debased by promiscuous and imprecise usage to describe virtually any form of repetitive behavior." Some of us, we are told, are "sex addicts," others are "TV addicts" or "shopaholics." The result is that it is no longer clear what it means to have an addiction. When the word is used in this loose, all-embracing way, most of us could be said to be "addicted" to something or other.

Nevertheless, there are some similarities between binge eating and the classic addictions involving alcohol and drug abuse, and many people focus on these similarities to support the addiction model of binge eating. They point out that whether the behavior is alcohol/drug abuse or binge eating, the person

- Has cravings or urges to engage in the behavior.
- Feels a loss of control over the behavior.
- Is preoccupied with thoughts about the behavior.
- Might use the behavior to relieve tension and negative feelings.
- Denies the severity of the problem.
- Attempts to keep the problem secret.
- Persists in the behavior despite its adverse effects.
- Often makes repeated unsuccessful attempts to stop.

These similarities are, however, partial. They are interesting, and some are relevant to treatment—for example, the use of the behavior to deal with tension—but the fact that things are similar or have properties in common does not make them the same.

> The fact that things are similar or have properties in common does not make them the same.

Moreover, focusing exclusively on the similarities, as is often done, neglects important differences between these forms of behavior, differences that are both central to the understanding of them and central to their successful treatment.

There are three main differences between binge eating and substance abuse, all of which are important:

1. Binge eating does not involve the consumption of a particular class of foods. Elsewhere Terence Wilson has pointed out that if bulimia nervosa were an addiction, patients should preferentially consume specific "addictive" foods. This is not the case in bulimia nervosa, and the same is true in binge eating disorder. The key eating abnormality in binge eating is the amount of food consumed, not what foods are eaten (as we discussed in Chapter 1).

2. Those who binge eat have a drive to avoid the behavior. People with binge eating problems, other than those with binge eating disorder, are continually trying to restrict their food intake, that is, they are attempting to diet. What distresses them about their binge eating is that it represents a failure to control their eating and carries the risk of weight gain. There is no phenomenon equivalent to dieting in alcohol (or drug) abuse. Those who abuse alcohol have no inherent drive to avoid alcohol against the background of which their excessive drinking takes place. In fact a major goal of addiction treatment programs is to instill in the addict the determination not to engage in the addictive behavior. In most binge eating problems, in contrast, this determination already exists in the form of the strong desire to control food intake. Indeed, the drive to control eating is a problem in its own right as it perpetuates the binge eating (as we discussed in Chapter 4).

3. Those who binge eat fear engaging in the behavior. In most binge eating problems, accompanying the drive to diet is a set of attitudes toward shape and weight characterized by the overevaluation of shape and weight (see Chapter 4). Self-worth is judged almost exclusively in terms of appearance and weight, and (as we discussed in Chapter 6) these attitudes play an important role in perpetuating the disorder through encouraging persistent and strict dieting. Once again, there is no equivalent phenomenon in alcohol or drug abuse. In other words, the desire to restrict eating encourages those with binge eating problems to binge. In contrast, those addicted to alcohol or drugs are not vulnerable to abuse of these substances as a result of their wish to avoid them.

As can be seen, there are markedly different mechanisms involved in binge eating and substance abuse and these point to two diametrically opposed approaches to their treatment. In the case of most binge eating problems, treatment needs to focus on moderating self-restraint. In contrast, treatments for addiction need to focus on strengthening it.

On the other hand, binge eating does occur among some people who do not diet particularly intensely, specifically many of those with binge eating disorder. The binge eating of these people is not driven by dieting, or at least to a far lesser degree. Difficulties coping with stress seem to be much more important. So, potentially, there is more of an overlap between the mechanisms driving their binge eating and those driving alcohol or drug abuse.

THE RELATIONSHIP BETWEEN BINGE EATING AND SUBSTANCE ABUSE

Even if binge eating is not itself an addiction, are the similarities between binge eating and substance abuse indicative of an association between the two? Could both problems be caused by a single underlying abnormality? To answer these questions, studies have been carried out to determine how often and under what circumstances the two problems appear in the same person or the same family.

Substance Abuse among People with Binge Eating Problems

While proponents of the addiction model of binge eating often state that the rates of alcohol and drug abuse are disproportionately high among those with binge eating problems, this is not the case. While research findings indicate that the rates are indeed raised, they are no higher than those among people with other psychiatric disorders.

Binge Eating Problems among Those with Substance Abuse

If there is a specific association between binge eating and substance abuse, those with alcohol and drug addiction should have a raised rate of binge eating problems. This does indeed appear to be the case, but once again it seems that is a nonspecific association in that there is an elevated rate of eating problems among people with other psychiatric disorders, for example, anxiety disorders and depression.

Family Studies

Several studies have reported a raised rate of substance abuse among the relatives of people with bulimia nervosa. This finding is interesting but, like the others already mentioned, difficult to interpret. The rates seem to be no higher than those among the relatives of people with other psychiatric disorders. This is not what would be expected if binge eating problems and substance abuse were the result of a common underlying process.

The Relationship between the Disorders over Time

To understand the relationship between two disorders, it is also important to know whether one tends to lead to the other or vice versa. Studies of those people with alcohol problems who also have an eating problem suggest that the latter develops first. This finding is not surprising, however, since eating problems typically begin at an earlier age than alcohol problems.

The Effects of Treatment

If a single abnormality underlies both binge eating problems and substance abuse, then the successful treatment of one of these problems might be expected to lead to the emergence of the other (unless the underlying abnormality had also been corrected). This phenomenon is sometimes referred to as *symptom substitution*. There is no evidence that it occurs in this context: indeed, there is evidence that it does not, at least among people with binge eating problems (see Box 12).

BOX 12. Changes in alcohol intake in those treated for an eating disorder.

It is commonly assumed that people who have both a binge eating problem and a high alcohol intake do less well in treatment. Sometimes voiced is the related concern that elimination of the binge eating problem might worsen the accompanying alcohol problem.

Data from a study of "enhanced cognitive behavior therapy" (CBT-E) were used to investigate these relationships. One hundred and forty-nine patients with an eating disorder were divided into two groups, a high-intake group whose weekly alcohol intake exceeded healthy guidelines and a low-intake group whose intake was within healthy limits. Both the low- and the high-intake groups suffered from an eating disorder of equivalent severity.

There were two main findings. First, the low and high alcohol intake groups responded in an almost identical way to CBT-E, thus refuting the assumption that those with a high alcohol intake would respond less well. Second, during treatment the alcohol intake of most patients in the high intake group fell to within healthy limits despite it not being a focus of CBT-E. The alcohol intake of a small minority did increase, but these people made limited progress in all respects so it does not appear that improvement in their eating problem was encouraging them to drink. In other words it seems that there was no symptom substitution.

Source: Karacic, M., Wales, J. A., Arcelus, J., Palmer, R. L., Cooper, Z., & Fairburn, C. G. (2011). Changes in alcohol intake in response to transdiagnostic cognitive behaviour therapy for eating disorders. *Behaviour Research and Therapy, 49,* 573–577.

THE IMPLICATIONS OF THE ADDICTION
MODEL FOR TREATMENT

Our goal is to abstain from compulsive overeating one day at a time. We do this through daily personal contact, meetings and by following the twelve-step program of Alcoholics Anonymous, changing only the words "alcohol" and "alcoholic" to "food" and "compulsive overeater."
—*Overeaters Anonymous leaflet*

Given that there are no grounds for claiming that binge eating is the result of an addictive process, is it appropriate to treat it as one? The straight answer is "No." The principles underlying addiction-oriented

The principles underlying addiction-oriented treatment are at total odds with the treatment that has proved most effective.

treatment are at total odds with the treatment approach that has proved most effective for binge eating problems.

Treatment, according to the addiction model, should be based on the approach used by Alcoholics Anonymous (and other related groups) for helping those with alcohol problems. This is the so-called "12-step" approach. Four features distinguish this approach from the most successful form of treatment for binge eating problems, a psychological treatment termed cognitive behavior therapy or CBT (described in Chapter 8):

1. Twelve-step approach: The disorder is an illness for which there is no cure. A book of daily readings for members of Overeaters Anonymous states, "*It is the experience of recovering compulsive overeaters that the illness is progressive. The disease does not get better; it gets worse. Even while we abstain, the illness progresses.*"

CBT approach: Recovery is well within the reach of most people. Long-term follow-up studies of bulimia nervosa and binge eating disorder indicate that full recovery is possible and not uncommon, and that with appropriate treatment the great majority of people improve substantially (see Chapter 8).

2. Twelve-step approach: Immediate abstinence is paramount. The focus of the 12-step approach is on stopping binge eating as rapidly as possible, and group pressure may be applied to serve this end. In some treatment meetings, abstinent participants are identified and praised, whereas those who have not been abstinent are given little or no opportunity to speak: indeed, they may be asked to leave.

CBT approach: Emphasis on the immediate cessation of binge eating is neither reasonable nor realistic. The abstinence stance is heartless and unreasonable. While with good advice and support many people can stop binge eating fairly rapidly, many others cannot. It may take them weeks or months to get to this point. The CBT approach places no emphasis on the immediate cessation of binge eating.

3. *Twelve-step approach: A major strategy for achieving abstinence from binge eating is an additional form of abstinence: the total lifelong avoidance of the ("toxic") foods that trigger binge eating.*

CBT approach: Food avoidance should be eliminated, not encouraged. As discussed earlier, the view that certain foods are toxic and somehow cause people to binge has no basis in fact. Clinical and experimental evidence indicate that it is the very attempts to avoid these foods that make many people vulnerable to binge (see Chapter 4). It is for this reason CBT focuses on eliminating food avoidance rather than encouraging it. The addiction model would predict that this would promote further binge eating. The research indicates that the exact opposite is the case.

4. *Twelve-step approach: One is either in control or out of control; foods are safe or toxic; one is abstinent or not.* Underpinning the abstinence approach is an all-or-nothing way of thinking.

CBT approach: Black-and-white thinking is a problem that needs to be addressed. To take one example, an all-or-nothing view of progress after treatment encourages people to regard any setback as a "relapse" rather than a "lapse." This way of thinking leads people to give up in the face of slips when there is no need for them to do so. All-or-nothing thinking is common among people who binge, and it seems to contribute to it, as we discussed in Chapter 4. So, rather than reinforcing this way of thinking, as in the abstinence approach, it is important to help people recognize and counter it.

There is, of course, more to addiction-based treatments than I have presented. Their greatest strength is the high level of long-term support and fellowship that many provide. This, combined with the simplicity of their message, makes them attractive to some people. However, the "bottom line" must be effectiveness. The 12-step approach to binge eating problems has never been evaluated properly, whereas a great deal is known about the effectiveness of other forms of treatment. These are the subject of the final chapter in this section of the book.

CHAPTER 8

The Treatment
of Binge Eating Problems

You have now learned what we know about binge eating problems—
how we define them; what types of psychological, social, and physical
factors are involved in causing them; and who, as far as the research
has been able to discern, is affected by them. You should also be
aware that what we do not know is substantial, perhaps especially in
the area of causation. It is now time for us to turn to the subject of
treatment, a topic about which much more is known.

This chapter summarizes current knowledge about the treatment
of binge eating problems. All the main forms of treatment are discussed, but particular emphasis is placed on the use of antidepressant
drugs and a specific short-term psychotherapy called cognitive behavior therapy—commonly abbreviated as CBT—as these approaches
have been the focus of particularly intense research efforts.

THE ROLE OF HOSPITALIZATION

One question that may occur to those of you whose binge eating
problem has persisted despite past attempts at treatment is whether
hospitalization is indicated. In fact, hospitalization is rarely appropriate. Both clinical and research experience indicate that the great

majority of people with binge eating problems may be successfully treated as outpatients.

Hospitalization may not only be unnecessary, it may be counterproductive. People tend to stop binge eating soon after being hospitalized, and it is therefore easy to draw the conclusion that hospitalization is helping them overcome their eating problem. In fact, however, people tend to stop binge eating because a hospital is a foreign environment where access to food is limited, because they are protected from many of the stresses of everyday life, and because privacy is limited. In reality their binge eating is merely in abeyance. It is likely to resume after discharge.

The best inpatient programs try to prevent relapse after discharge by helping people develop skills for dealing with the processes that lead them to binge. The trouble is that the hospital environment is not a good place in which to do this. The therapist and the patient need to tackle the binge eating problem as it normally exists, that is, in the outside world.

Of course, there are circumstances under which admission to a hospital is advisable. Three stand out:

1. Some people are suicidal and so need the protection of a hospital.
2. Some people's physical health is a cause for concern (see Chapter 5).
3. Hospitalization may also be indicated if the eating problem has not responded to well-delivered outpatient treatment.

In practice, these circumstances apply to less than 5% of cases. There is, however, one other reason for considering hospitalization. Namely, in countries without socialized health care, insurance coverage may provide the only viable means of paying for treatment, and some insurance policies only cover inpatient care. Under these circumstances, people have little choice other than to be hospitalized.

Whatever the reason for hospitalization, it should always be viewed as a preliminary to good outpatient treatment.

ANTIDEPRESSANT MEDICATION AND OTHER FORMS OF DRUG TREATMENT

Interest in using antidepressant drugs to treat binge eating problems began in 1982 with the publication of two scientific papers describing a favorable response in patients with bulimia nervosa. Since then, much research has been conducted, and the facts have become clearer.

Within a few weeks of treatment with antidepressant medication there is, on average, a 50 to 60% reduction in the frequency of binge eating. People report experiencing a reduced urge to binge. Associated with this reduction is an equivalent fall in the frequency of any associated self-induced vomiting, an improvement in mood and sense of control over eating, and decreased preoccupation with eating. These effects occur whether or not the person is depressed, but they tend not to last, whether or not the person continues to take the medication.

Research has also shown that antidepressant drugs have a selective effect on eating habits: the binge eating is affected but any accompanying dieting is not. It is likely that the persistence of dieting explains why these benefits of antidepressant medication tend not to last.

Awareness that antidepressant drugs are of limited value in the longer term has led to decreased enthusiasm for their use. However, they are still employed as a treatment for any accompanying clinical depression, and they can be extremely effective in this regard.

What about other drugs? The effects of mood stabilizing drugs such as lithium, drugs used for epilepsy, and appetite suppressants have all been studied, but none is promising. At present there is no accepted drug treatment for binge eating problems.

COGNITIVE BEHAVIOR THERAPY

In marked contrast to the research on antidepressant medication, that on psychological treatments has confirmed that they can be of considerable help. The most effective treatment is a specific form of CBT that I developed when I was training to be a psychiatrist in Edinburgh. Originally, the treatment was designed for people with bulimia nervosa but it has since been modified to make it suitable for any type of binge eating problem.

CBT is well suited to the treatment of binge eating problems because its cognitive elements address the cognitive aspects of these problems—the overevaluation of shape and weight, the dietary rules, and the all-or-nothing thinking—while its behavioral components tackle the disturbed eating habits. Its core characteristics are listed in Table 7.

CBT addresses the binge eating problem in a systematic manner by using a carefully planned sequence of interventions designed to fit the needs of the individual. It begins with the use of behavioral and educational techniques to help the person regain control over his or her eating, a key element being establishing a pattern of regular eating. This is crucial because it tends to displace most binges. However, the improvement that results is fragile because most people remain vulnerable to further episodes of binge eating. Therefore, in the second stage of the treatment the emphasis switches to reducing this vulnerability by tackling any tendency to diet and the use of binge eating to cope with adverse events and moods. The third stage focuses on maintaining the changes made and minimizing the risk of relapse.

CBT has been very extensively researched. It has been tested in studies in the United States, Canada, the United Kingdom, other countries in Europe, and in Australia and New Zealand. No other treatment for binge eating problems has equivalent support. It has also been compared with a wide range of other treatments, both pharmacological and psychological, and no treatment has been found to be as effective. Recently, in a uniquely demanding test of the latest version of CBT, so-called "enhanced CBT" or CBT-E (described later), Stig Poulsen and Susanne Lunn from Copenhagen compared 20 sessions of CBT (given over 20 weeks) with 100 sessions of psychoanalytic psychotherapy (given over 2 years). CBT-E was clearly superior, both after 20 weeks and after 2 years.

Overall, the research findings indicate that CBT has a rapid

TABLE 7. The core characteristics of the cognitive behavioral approach.

Format

Typically about 20 one-to-one treatment sessions over 20 weeks with the sessions being twice weekly at first.

Structure and Content

Stage One

- Creating a "formulation"—a diagram representing the main processes that appear to be maintaining the eating problem. This greatly facilitates change.

- Recording in detail all eating and drinking at the time that it occurs, together with relevant thoughts and feelings.

- Introducing a pattern of regular eating. This displaces most binges.

- Developing the ability to resist urges to binge.

- Receiving personalized education about food, eating, shape, and weight.

Stage Two

- Addressing concerns about shape and weight as well as shape checking, shape avoidance, and feeling fat.

- Introducing avoided foods into the diet and gradually eliminating other forms of dieting.

- Developing skills for dealing with day-to-day difficulties that might otherwise trigger binges

Stage Three

- Developing means of minimizing the risk of relapse

Adapted from Fairburn, C. G. (2008). *Cognitive behavior therapy and eating disorders.* New York: Guilford Press.

effect on binge eating. This effect is greater in magnitude than that obtained with antidepressant drugs and it persists in most cases. In common with antidepressant medication, it is accompanied by improvements in mood, concentration, and sense of control over eating. In addition, the tendency to diet decreases and concerns about shape and weight wane. These latter two effects are likely to explain why the effects of CBT tend to be enduring.

OTHER PSYCHOLOGICAL TREATMENTS

It is sometimes claimed that all psychological treatments are equally effective. This is quite untrue. Some psychological treatments have little or no impact on binge eating problems.

This said, two psychological treatments other than CBT have been shown to have consistent effects, albeit not as great as those obtained with CBT. These are interpersonal psychotherapy and "guided self-help," a streamlined form of CBT.

Interpersonal Psychotherapy

Interpersonal psychotherapy (or IPT) is a short-term psychotherapy that focuses on helping people to improve their relationships with other people. While it was originally developed as a treatment for depression, it also helps many people with binge eating problems. How it works is uncertain, but it is certainly true that many people with binge eating problems have problematic relationships, as we discussed in Chapter 4.

When used to treat bulimia nervosa, IPT has been found to be as effective as CBT but much slower to work. The new version of CBT, CBT-E, appears to be clearly superior to IPT. The one eating disorder in which IPT may have a role is binge eating disorder, possibly because of the important role interpersonal difficulties play in triggering these people's binges. This said, guided self-help is about as effective and much more straightforward to implement.

Guided Self-Help

Guided self-help is a streamlined form of CBT. I developed this treatment at Oxford University together with my colleague Jacqueline Carter (who has since returned to Canada). The idea of developing a simpler form of CBT sprang from the observation that a subgroup of people with binge eating problems respond rapidly and easily to CBT without much input from a therapist. It seemed that these people were able to treat themselves using CBT principles. What we therefore did was create a self-help program based upon CBT and this was published in the original edition of *Overcoming Binge Eating*. Part II of this book consists of an extensively revised version of the program based upon CBT-E.

The original self-help program concentrated mainly on helping people improve their eating habits. It consisted of the behavioral and educational components of CBT but it had none of the more complex cognitive elements, so it was simpler than full CBT. The program was designed to be used in two ways:

1. *Pure self-help.* Use of the program on its own with no external support.
2. *Guided self-help.* Use of the program with external support. The support need not be from highly trained therapists, as their role is confined to helping the person make the best possible use of the self-help program. Thus this is a "program-led" treatment rather than a "therapist-led" one.

These two forms of self-help have been extensively studied. The main findings are summarized below:

1. *Overcoming Binge Eating* is the best studied of the self-help programs for

   > Overcoming Binge Eating *is the best studied self-help program.*

   binge eating problems. Indeed, it is probably the best studied self-help program of any type.
2. In general, guided self-help is more effective than pure self-help, although some people are able to treat themselves.
3. Guided self-help is remarkably effective as a treatment for binge eating disorder and related states (e.g., see Box 13).
4. There has been less research on the use of guided self-help in the treatment of bulimia nervosa and the atypical eating disorders, and the findings are somewhat inconsistent. This said, it is clear that it is effective in substantial numbers of cases.

Guided self-help has many advantages over more conventional forms of therapy. These include being relatively inexpensive and more readily accessed as it does not require a highly trained thera-

---

BOX 13. Guided self-help for recurrent binge eating.

One hundred and twenty-three patients with recurrent binge eating (mostly fulfilling the diagnosis binge eating disorder) were randomly allocated to receive either guided self-help or the usual treatment provided by a health maintenance organization (HMO). Guided self-help involved following the program in the original edition of *Overcoming Binge Eating* supported by eight 25-minute sessions from a junior "therapist" given over 12 weeks. The patients were assessed before treatment, and 6 and 12 months after completing treatment.

Compared to the HMO's usual forms of treatment, more of those who received guided self-help stopped binge eating (64 vs. 45%), despite the brevity and simplicity of the intervention. They also reported greater improvements in dieting, shape and weight concerns, and depression.

Source: Striegel-Moore, R. H., Wilson, G. T., DeBar, L., Perrin, N., Lynch, F., Rosselli, F., & Kraemer, H. C. (2010). Cognitive behavioral guided self-help for the treatment of recurrent binge eating. *Journal of Consulting and Clinical Psychology, 78,* 312–321.

---

pist. Pure self-help has yet further advantages as it totally sidesteps some of the barriers to obtaining treatment, including cost, absence of local treatment resources, and difficulty attending appointments. In addition, pure self-help allows people to receive "treatment" at a time, place, and pace that suits them. Last, but not least, it has the advantage of being inherently empowering. Overall, both forms of self-help have much to commend them.

WHEN TO USE SELF-HELP

What conclusions can we draw from the research on the treatment of binge eating problems, and where does self-help fit in?

The most important point to emphasize is that if you, or someone you know, is seeking professional help for a binge eating problem, the treatment of choice is CBT on a one-to-one basis and, ideally, CBT-E. (The website *www.credo-oxford.com* provides up-to-date information on the treatment.) Most people benefit substantially, and in the majority of cases the changes last. It must be stressed, however, that some people do not improve or they make only limited gains. These people need additional help. On the other hand, substantial numbers respond to simpler approaches, such as pure or guided self-help.

Given the research findings, a "stepped care" approach to treatment delivery seems sensible with a simple treatment being used first, and with more complex ones only being employed if the simple one proves ineffective. Thus, in the case of recurrent binge eating, the two steps are as follows:

- *Step 1.* Self-help (guided or pure)
- *Step 2.* One-to-one therapy, ideally CBT or CBT-E

This strategy is evidence-based and applies across all types of binge eating problem unless you are underweight. If you are underweight (i.e., have a BMI below 18.5; see "Getting Ready," Table 8, p. 125), you should seek professional advice because self-help on its own is unlikely to be sufficient.

WHY USE THIS SELF-HELP PROGRAM?

Why use the self-help program in Part II? There are two reasons. First, as mentioned already, the original self-help program published in *Overcoming Binge Eating* is the best tested program available. Second, the new version of the program takes account of advances in the understanding of binge eating problems, advances that have been reflected in the development of the "enhanced" version of CBT, CBT-E. CBT-E includes a new way of conceptualizing eating problems, improved ways of regaining control over eating, a more sophisticated approach to the addressing of concerns about shape and weight, and much more emphasis on relapse prevention. The self-help program in Part II is, in essence, a self-help version of CBT-E.

PART II

An Enhanced Self-Help Program for Those Who Binge[1]

[1]Copyright 2013 by Christopher G. Fairburn. Both the original version of this program and this new enhanced version were developed with the support of the Wellcome Trust.

Getting Ready

I read the program from beginning to end and knew immediately that it made so much sense. I underlined point after point. It didn't simply say "Eat this" and "Avoid that." Rather, it explained how to get on the right track in a realistic step-by-step way. I felt inspired because it understood my problem. It was exactly what I was looking for and exactly what I needed.

No self-help program will be successful unless the person undertaking it genuinely wants to change. So this is where we should start. And even if you are certain you want to change, I suggest you read this section because it will encourage you still further.

WHY CHANGE?

As I grow into middle age I realize with great sadness how much energy I have directed toward controlling my weight and eating, and the misery of the regular and consequent binges. I could be doing something productive with my energy—building relationships, reading, writing. I don't know what I might do, but I don't want my epitaph to be "Jane wished she was thin." It was this, in the end, that made me decide to change.

By this point in the book you should be sure, if you were not already, whether you binge. If you do binge, the key issue is whether you want to change. Do you want to stop binge eating? It is certainly possible to change: It is possible to start eating normally again; possible to enjoy eating rather than eating with regret and guilt; possible to be happy eating with others.

As we discussed in Part I, how severely, if at all, binge eating affects a person's life varies greatly from person to person. Only you can decide how pressing the need is for change. Because your motivation is likely to wax and wane, it often helps to have a stable set of guidelines by which you can judge the benefits of change, unaffected by fluctuations in the severity of your eating problem. Furthermore, if you have a long history of binge eating, it is possible that you have adjusted your life to accommodate the problem. If so, you need to consider whether this is the right thing to be doing.

The Advantages of Attempting to Change

One of my difficulties in deciding to change was that it seemed self-indulgent. After all, lots of people have problems with their eating and weight. But the truth I had to face was that the problem was so much more invasive than it seemed—it affected everything. I couldn't be me while I still had the problem.

Start by drawing up a list of the potential advantages of change. To help you do so, ask yourself the following questions:

If I stop binge eating . . .
- *Will I feel better about myself?*
- *Will it improve my quality of life?*
- *Will my physical health be enhanced?*
- *Will others benefit?*

People are often surprised at how much better they feel once they stop binge eating. Even minor binge eating problems can have subtle adverse effects on many aspects of

People are often surprised at how much better they feel once they stop binge eating.

life. You may be unnecessarily irritable at times, your concentration may not be as good as it could be, you may avoid social events that you would like to attend (see Chapter 4), and your physical health may be impaired (see Chapter 5). Perhaps you don't realize that these are direct results of your binge eating problem and will resolve as it improves. Another benefit of change is the effect it has on morale and self-image: many people find it restores their sense of self-respect and self-worth. As I mentioned in Chapter 4, one of the most gratifying aspects of helping people overcome binge eating problems is seeing the person underneath emerge as the problem recedes. The depression, tension, and irritability fade, concentration improves, and old interests (perhaps forgotten) return.

It is also important to take a longer term perspective. I suggest you look again at the quote on page 119. Basically, Jane didn't want to waste her life. With this in mind, ask yourself the following four questions:

How many years have I spent binge eating?
How much time has it taken up?
How much money have I unnecessarily spent?
Have I been adjusting my life around my binge eating?

And, of course, you would be in a better position to control your weight if you had control over your eating.

> *You would be in a better position to control your weight if you had control over your eating.*

For some people one of the most compelling reasons to stop binge eating is to put a halt to the harm that self-induced vomiting and laxative abuse may be doing to their health. When you stop doing these things, you can expect a gradual return of normal sensations of fullness and hunger, an increase in energy, and an improvement in your overall sense of wellbeing.

The other people in your life—friends, family, and coworkers—will also benefit if you regain control over your eating. You will stop being unpredictably irritable and moody; you will be less touchy about eating and less sensitive about your shape and weight; and you will be happier being with others. And you will have more time—for yourself, for work, and for other people. As a result, your relationships and your work performance will improve.

The Disadvantages of Attempting to Change

Having compiled your list of reasons to change, you should think of possible disadvantages. There may be some, and it is worth balancing these against the advantages. How would you feel if you did not succeed? Perhaps you are tempted to do nothing rather than risk failure. While this stance is understandable, it is best resisted. There is every reason to expect that, with the right sort of help, your binge eating problem will improve, if not resolve altogether. Furthermore, if you decide to use this self-help program and make a determined effort to do so, there can be no question of failure. If things do not improve, the program simply was not right for you; it will have failed, not you. And if that is the case, there are many other options available, as we are about to discuss.

One other point to note is that a good way of assessing the seriousness of a problem is to see how easy it is to overcome. If you discover that you can readily stop binge eating, then at least you have learned that the problem is surmountable. On the other hand, if you discover that it is not easy to change, you will have learned that it is a significant problem, perhaps more so than you thought. In this case you should perhaps consider taking it more seriously than you have been doing.

HOW TO CHANGE: THE VARIOUS OPTIONS

Assuming you have decided to tackle your binge eating problem, what should you do? We considered the main options in Chapter 8. In principle, there are four.

1. **Seek professional help.** There are many professionals who help people who have binge eating problems. They include

psychologists, psychiatrists, general physicians, dietitians, social workers, nurses, and others. Some specialize in the area. Guidance on how to find a local specialist is given in Appendix I.

2. *Join a self-help group.* Many such groups are excellent, but unfortunately some are not. Some have questionable views on binge eating problems and how they should be tackled. Also, some are focused more on helping people live with their problem than overcoming it. Before committing yourself to a self-help group, find out as much as you can about it. If you do decide to join one, see if it suits you. Remember, you can always leave if the group isn't right for you.

3. *Use this self-help program.* Whether you are male or female, single or married, living alone or with others, you can use this self-help program. You should reject this program only if one of the exclusion criteria mentioned later applies.

4. *Combine professional help and self-help.* There are two ways to do this. You can use this program on your own while at the same time receiving therapy of some other sort—therapy directed at, for example, self-esteem or relationships. This is a good plan so long as you have discussed it with your therapist. He or she must be fully informed in case there is a clash between this program and the help being provided.

   The other way of combining self-help and professional help is what was referred to as "guided self-help" in Chapter 8. It involves following the program with the support and guidance of a therapist. In this case the therapist (the terms *facilitator, guide,* or *coach* are sometimes used) helps you monitor your progress, provides encouragement, and guides you in identifying solutions to problems that you encounter on the way.

Deciding Which Option Is Best for You

If you think you need professional help, it is important that you take steps to obtain it. This self-help program must not divert you from doing so.

However, this program, used with or without professional help, is likely to be appropriate for most people with a binge eating problem. Having said this, I must stress that overcoming a binge eating problem is not easy; it generally requires a lot of effort. Half-hearted attempts tend not to succeed. I therefore urge you to suspend any doubts about the program—after all, it is strongly evidence-based— and do your very best to follow it.

WHEN TO START

If you have decided to change but hesitate to commit yourself, the best advice is to take the plunge and get started. There is one point to note, however, and it applies to most forms of help but especially to this program: if you can foresee that major distractions are likely to get in the way, it is best to delay starting. If you are about to relocate, change jobs, get married, have a baby, or go on vacation, postpone starting until the distraction has passed or at least its influence has waned.

To get the most out of the program you will need at least a couple of months free from significant distractions. Anything less will not be enough.

WHEN SELF-HELP MAY NOT
BE APPROPRIATE

You should not use this program if any of the following circumstances apply.

> *If you are underweight.* If your BMI (see Box 3, p. 26) is below
> 18.5, your weight is low. Table 8 shows what weights in
> pounds (for different heights) are equivalent to a BMI 18.5.
> If you weigh less than the weight shown for your height, you
> should not follow this program unless advised to do so by a
> therapist who is knowledgeable about eating problems (see

TABLE 8. Are you underweight?

Below is a table listing weights for different heights. Each weight represents a body mass index of 18.5. The figures apply to men and women between the ages of 18 and 60 years. To determine whether you are underweight, find your height on the table and look across at the weight for that height. If you weigh less than this weight, your body mass index is below 18.5. (If you use units other than feet, inches, and pounds, refer to the table in Appendix II to find out your BMI or use one of the many BMI calculators on the Internet.)

Height[a] (feet, inches)	Weight[b] (pounds)	Height[a] (feet, inches)	Weight[b] (pounds)
4'10"	89	5'8"	122
4'10½"	90	5'8½"	124
4'11"	92	5'9"	125
4'11½"	93	5'9½"	127
5'0"	95	5'10"	129
5'½"	97	5'10½"	131
5'1"	98	5'11"	133
5'1½"	100	5'11½"	135
5'2"	101	6'0"	137
5'2½"	103	6'½"	138
5'3"	105	6'1"	142
5'3½"	106	6'1½"	143
5'4"	108	6'2"	144
5'4½"	110	6'2½"	146
5'5"	111	6'3"	148
5'5½"	113	6'3½"	150
5'6"	115	6'4"	152
5'6½"	117	6'4½"	154
5'7"	118	6'5"	156
5'7½"	120	6'5½"	158

[a]Without shoes; [b]without shoes, light indoor clothing.

Appendix I). On its own, the program is unlikely to help if you are underweight.

If you have a serious physical illness. If you have a physical illness that might be affected by a change in your eating habits, you should use this program only under the supervision of a physician. This advice applies particularly to those with diabetes.

If you are pregnant. Women who are pregnant should not use the program without first discussing the matter with their obstetrician.

If you suspect that your physical health is being affected by the binge eating problem (see Chapter 5). If this applies, you should consult a physician to have your health checked before embarking on the program. Once you have done so and have informed the physician of your plan, it may well be appropriate to embark upon the program.

If you are significantly depressed or demoralized. If you are feeling this way, you may not be able to summon up enough mental energy and optimism to make good use of the program. Under these circumstances seek the advice of a health professional and when doing so mention your binge eating problem. Once your mood has improved, you might well benefit from the program.

If you have a significant problem with alcohol, drugs, or repeated self-harm. If this is the case, it is best to seek professional help since this program on its own is unlikely to be sufficient.

WHAT WILL HAPPEN TO MY WEIGHT?

As we discussed in Chapter 4, most people with binge eating problems are highly concerned about their appearance and weight. It is therefore likely that you want to know what will happen to your weight if you follow the program. The answer is that there is generally little or no change. The reasons for this were explained in Chapter 5

(p. 72). However, some people lose weight and others gain, and it is impossible to predict what will happen in any individual case. If your weight is low as a result of your own efforts, you are likely to need to gain some weight because continuing to diet is rarely compatible with overcoming a binge eating problem. On the other hand, if you are medically overweight (see Box 3, p. 26, and Appendix II), it is less easy to predict what will happen, although you are most unlikely to gain weight.

At this stage I suggest that you concentrate your efforts on overcoming your binge eating problem and accept for the meantime whatever change in weight that occurs. If this seems too difficult, try putting aside the question of your weight for, say, a month while embarking on the program. Then, after the month has passed, take stock and evaluate your progress in terms of your eating and your weight. By this point you will be in a much better position to decide whether to focus on your binge eating problem or your weight.

It is, of course, entirely appropriate to monitor your weight as you progress through the program. Advice on how to do this is given in Step 1.

HOW TO USE THE PROGRAM

The program is comprised of a series of "steps" and, as in the cognitive behavioral treatment on which it is based, the steps are additive, that is, each step

> *Start at the beginning and work your way through to the end. It is not a good idea to skip steps or do bits of this or that.*

builds upon the previous one. It is therefore not a good idea to dip around in the program, doing bits of this and bits of that. Instead, you should start at the beginning and work your way through to the end, following the guidelines provided . . . *but before doing that it is most important that you read Chapters 1, 4, and 5 of Part I of this book.* The program assumes that you have read these chapters.

> *It is essential that you first read Chapters 1, 4, and 5.*

This said, it is likely that some elements of the program will not be relevant to you. The program has been designed for all those

Not all of the program will be relevant to you.

who binge eat and, as explained in Part I, binge eating problems vary in their nature and severity. Most people who binge also diet, often strictly, but some do not diet at all. Similarly, some are highly concerned about their appearance and weight, while others are not. Some are perfectionists, and meticulously organized, whereas others are on the chaotic side. And some vomit, or take laxatives or diuretics, whereas others do not. As explained in Chapter 4, all these characteristics contribute in their own way to the persistence of the binge eating problem and therefore need to be addressed by the program. For this reason, the program has multiple components, and some may not apply to you. For the most part it will be obvious what applies and what does not. But if you are in doubt, the best policy is to assume that the advice does apply and follow it.

Some Tips to Help You Succeed

Persevere, especially when the advice is difficult to follow. In general, the harder you find it to follow the advice, the more important it is that you do

The harder you find it to follow the advice, the more important it is to do so.

so. When things are difficult it is often because you are now directly tackling the most powerful processes maintaining your binge eating problem.

Keep in mind that you will not need to follow the program forever. You will need to do many things to break out of your binge eating problem but only some will need to be kept up over the long term. These differ from person to person and will be identified toward the end of the program.

Do not rush through the program. Instead, proceed at the pace suggested since experience indicates that this rate works best. Sometimes it is a good idea to stay at a step for an extra week or so to see if there is more that you can do. And if you have a setback, it is often wise to go back a step in the program.

In general, it takes people between 4 and 6 months to work through the program.

In general, it takes people between 4 and 6 months to work through the program and get the most out of it. Some people are able to change rapidly; for others it is a slow process. The key issue is whether you are making progress. If you are moving in the right direction, then it is reasonable to carry on. However, if you have not benefited by the time you have reached Step 5, you should seek outside help. The same applies if you get stuck on a step.

Do not expect overnight success. Do not be disappointed by less-than-dramatic results. Change takes time, and binge eating problems are not likely to resolve within just a few weeks.

Do not expect to make smooth and steady progress. It is normal for progress to occur in fits and starts. There are likely to be times when things go well, times when you get stuck, and times when you have setbacks and the problem seems to worsen. In the course of the program, you will be monitoring your progress. This will allow you to identify, and tackle, any obstacles that are getting in the way.

Do not expect the urge to binge to disappear as soon as you stop binge eating. Even after you have completely stopped binge eating, you will intermittently experience urges to binge. These urges will persist for some months. Don't be discouraged by this. These urges will be triggered by the same circumstances that used to trigger actual binges. The program will help you resist these urges, and gradually they will fade away.

Be sure to hold weekly review sessions. Integral to the program are regular "review sessions" in which you assess your progress.

Integral to the program are regular "review sessions."

Until your binge eating is well under control, have two of these review sessions a week. Thereafter they can be weekly. It is a good idea to book them in advance and view them as equivalent to an appointment with a therapist, but in this case you are your own therapist. Try to set aside 15 to 30 minutes for these sessions. They are important, and you should not allow other activities to take precedence over them. (Guidelines for conducting the review sessions are provided at the end of each step.)

Consider enlisting someone to help you. While many people use the program on their own, others enlist outside help. Helpers are of two types, and their roles differ. You might choose a friend or relative. In this case their main role is to provide support and encouragement at times of difficulty. Helpers of this type need to remain in the background unless their assistance is requested. Alternatively, you may seek the help of a therapist with whom you have a professional rather than a personal relationship. Therapists can take a more active role than friends or relatives. Indeed, they can oversee your use of the program along the lines outlined in Chapter 8 (p. 113). Both types of helper need to familiarize themselves with the program if they are to support your use of it. (Appendix V provides guidelines for relatives and friends, and Appendix VI is for therapists.)

STEP 1

Starting Well

Step 1: Starting Well
Self-monitoring
Weekly weighing

Step 2: Regular Eating
Establishing a pattern of regular eating
Stopping vomiting and misusing laxatives or diuretics

Step 3: Alternatives to Binge Eating
Substituting alternative activities
Identifying changes in weight

Step 4: Problem Solving
Practicing problem solving

Step 5: Taking Stock
Reviewing progress
Deciding what else needs to be tackled

Dieting Module
Tackling strict
dieting

Body Image Module
Addressing shape concerns, shape
checking, shape avoidance, and feeling fat

Ending Well
Maintaining progress
Addressing setbacks

The program assumes you are familiar with the information in Chapters 1, 4, and 5.

You are now ready to start the program. But before doing so, remember that the program assumes you are familiar with the information in Chapters 1, 4, and 5 of the book. Do refresh your memory of them. This is important. Having done this you are ready to embark upon Step 1 which has two components, self-monitoring and weekly weighing.

STARTING SELF-MONITORING

Self-monitoring is central to the program. It serves two essential purposes:

1. *Monitoring provides you with important information about your eating problem.* You may say that you are all too aware of the problem and in a sense, of course, this is true. But accurate monitoring almost always highlights features that were not obvious to you beforehand. Monitoring gives you answers to these questions:

> Exactly what do I eat during my binges? How does it compare with what I eat at other times? Do my binges consist of foods that I am trying to avoid eating?
>
> Exactly when do my binges occur? Is there a predictable pattern? For example, do they always occur in the evening? Are weekdays different from weekends?
>
> Are there any triggers for my binges? Do my binges tend to occur under certain circumstances? Do they occur when I am bored, depressed, lonely, or anxious?
>
> Do my binges appear to serve any function? For example, do they relieve feelings of tension? Are they a way of punishing myself?

For reasons that I will explain later, you need answers to these questions to overcome your binge eating problem.

2. Monitoring also helps you change. When done properly, monitoring also helps people change. Monitoring your eating accurately *and at the time you are doing it* will gradually reveal that apparently automatic, out-of-control behavior is nothing of the sort. You do not have to binge whenever you feel tense or angry, or whenever you break one of your dietary rules. You have just grown so used to doing this that doing anything else seems impossible. Monitoring along the lines recommended will show you that you have options other than binge eating. Monitoring will help you change.

Why You Should Monitor, Despite Any Reservations

You may find yourself reluctant to monitor. Perhaps you have one or more of these reservations.

> *I have kept food records before, and it did not help.* It is most unlikely that you have monitored in the way recommended by this program. Give it a good try and see what happens.
>
> *Monitoring sounds like too much of a chore.* You may feel that you are too busy or that your lifestyle makes it impossible to monitor. It is certainly true that monitoring is demanding in terms of time and effort, but I have never encountered anyone whose lifestyle made it truly impossible to monitor. Your willingness to monitor is a test of your commitment to change.
>
> *I am too embarrassed about my eating to monitor.* If you feel like this, monitoring may indeed be particularly difficult. Nevertheless, if you are to overcome your binge eating problem, you have no alternative but to face up to it, and monitoring is the first step. Perhaps it helps to know that it will become second nature within a few weeks.
>
> *Monitoring will make me even more preoccupied with my eating.* This is true, but only in the short term (for a matter of weeks). The effect rapidly fades. And in any case the preoccupation is constructive because it focuses you on how to overcome your binge eating problem.

How to Use the Monitoring Records

A blank monitoring record is shown in Figure 15. You may download a copy from the *www.credo-oxford.com* website. You will need a fresh record for each day, and you will need to carry it with you wherever you go. You may be tempted to record your eating by using your smart phone or some other electronic device. This is not a good idea. When using devices of this type people note what and when they eat, but they tend not to record other important matters such as the circumstances at the time and any accompanying thoughts and feelings. Instructions for completing the monitoring records are given in Table 9.

Figure 16 shows a monitoring record completed by a woman with bulimia nervosa. You can see that she ate almost nothing until the evening, when she had a large binge. Figure 17 shows a record from someone with binge eating disorder. It shows the typical overeating upon which binge eating is superimposed.

Starting Self-Monitoring: What to Do

Start monitoring just as described, but do not try to change your eating just yet. It is important to begin the program by getting into the swing of accurate monitoring. You will be changing your eating in Step 2. Monitoring will need to become a habit since you will be doing it for the duration of the program. Do not take days off from monitoring (or from the program itself) and make sure not to omit binges from your records. This may be difficult, but it is essential that you are honest with yourself. To overcome a binge eating problem you need to confront the whole problem, and not a sanitized version of it.

Keep your monitoring records somewhere private and keep them all together so that you can look back over them. Reviewing your records will allow you to detect changes over time. (If you are using the guided self-help approach described earlier, you will need to review your monitoring records with your therapist.)

So, begin the program by monitoring until your first review session in 3 or 4 days' time. This will be described shortly.

Day				Date		
Time	Food and drink consumed	Place	*	V/L	Context and comments	

FIGURE 15. A blank monitoring record. An enlarged version of this figure may be downloaded from *www.credo-oxford.com*.

TABLE 9. Instructions for completing the monitoring records.

Do your best to be accurate and record things as closely as possible to the time when they occurred. In other words, try to record in "real time."

Column 1: Note here the time when you ate or drank anything.

Column 2: Record exactly what you ate and drank, including everything consumed in binges. Leave nothing out. Do not record calories. Instead, write down a simple description of what you ate and drank, and do so as soon as possible afterwards, preferably immediately. Trying to recall what you ate or drank some hours earlier is unreliable and will not help you change. For example, if you are out for a meal, it is a good idea to record between courses, perhaps by briefly popping outside to get some privacy. Only in this way will monitoring help you change your behavior. Also in column 2 identify with brackets those episodes of eating that you view as "meals." Do not bracket snacks or other episodes of eating.

Column 3: Specify where you were when you consumed the food or drink. If in your home, specify the room.

Column 4: Place an asterisk in this column opposite the food that you felt at the time was excessive. Binges will therefore be distinguished by a chain of asterisks.

Column 5: Use the V/L column to record when you vomit or misuse laxatives or diuretics.

Column 6: Use this column somewhat like a diary to note anything that seems to be influencing your eating. For example, whenever you put an asterisk in column 4, you should record in column 6 the circumstances at the time, the purpose being to identify the triggers of each episode of "excessive" eating. Perhaps you had just had an argument with someone and were angry. Or you may have been under social pressure to eat. Also use column 6 to record your weight each time you weigh yourself.

ESTABLISHING WEEKLY WEIGHING

Most people with binge eating problems are concerned about their weight, that is, the number on the scale, and often this is a major concern. Knowing their weight may be very important to them. As we discussed in Chapter 4, many go through a period of weighing themselves frequently, in some cases many times a day. However, weighing as often as this can become intolerable, and consequently

Day _Tuesday_   Date _June 18th_

Time	Food and drink consumed	Place	*	V/L	Context and comments
6:30	Black coffee Glass of water	Bedroom			Sleepless night. Feel gross and fat.
11:45	Black coffee 2 glasses of water	Staff room			Will not binge today! Starting to feel hungry so had an extra glass of water.
2:15	1 medium bottle diet coke ½ donut	Staff room			Ohh! Why do they ALWAYS have donuts? Only had half though, so it's OK.
3:30	4 donuts	Staff bathroom	*		Why do I do this? Couldn't help myself but did not want anyone to see me. Feel horrible and fat.
6:15	1 medium bottle of diet coke Glass of water	Kitchen			Am not going to eat again today
9:30	Pita bread and hummus 3 cinnamon raisin bagels 6 spoons of peanut butter 15 Oreo cookies ½ gallon vanilla ice cream 3 handfuls of nuts Large bottle of diet coke	Bedroom	* * * * * *	 V V	Am disgusted with myself. I have no willpower. Feel desperately alone. Going to bed early to stop any further eating.

FIGURE 16. A monitoring record completed by someone with bulimia nervosa.

Day _Thursday_   Date _April 20th_

Time	Food and drink consumed	Place	*	V/L	Context and comments
8:10	Plain bagel, butter ⎫ Decaf ⎭	Kitchen			
8:25	Half bagel, butter Decaf	Kitchen	*		Great bagel, but . . .
10:20	1 raisin muffin Decaf	At desk			Thinking about eating all morning
12:00	Medium pizza— pepperoni ⎫ Large diet coke ⎭	Staff cafeteria			Feel somewhat sick. Really full. I'm enormous.
3:00	2 donuts Decaf 2 donuts	At desk	* *		Must stop buying these. They are too good!

6:30	Large bag potato chips
	Diet coke
	2 plain bagels with
	   peanut butter
	Large slice chocolate
	   cake
	Diet coke
		Kitchen—
		standing
			*
			
			*
			
			*
					Tiresome drive home.
					Restless. I've nothing
					to do . . . just
					started eating . . .
					mindlessly. Enjoyed
					it at first.

7:15	3 KitKats Decaf tea 6 scoops chocolate ice cream 1 Cherry yogurt	Kitchen	* * *		I've started again. This is hopeless. I've no self-control.
9:00	2 decaf tea				

FIGURE 17. A monitoring record completed by someone with binge eating disorder.

some switch over to not weighing at all while remaining highly concerned about their weight.

As a result of following this program, your eating habits will change. You will therefore want to know what is happening to your weight. You may be afraid to find out, but avoiding knowing is a bad idea—you are left with your worst fears and no information. It is far better to monitor your weight as you progress through the program. The best way to do this is to weigh yourself once each week. Do not pay too much attention to individual readings since, as we discussed in Chapter 5 (p. 66), body weight fluctuates from day to day, and even within the day, in ways that are independent of changes in body fat. Individual readings on the scale can therefore be misleading as you may have hit a peak or trough in your weight fluctuations. Instead, you should look for trends over time, the minimum time period being several weeks (i.e., three or four individual weekly weight readings) because only in this way will you be able to distinguish genuine changes in weight from the day-to-day fluctuations taking place in the background.

A good way of identifying changes in your weight is to plot each reading onto a weight graph. Figure 18 shows the weight graph of a woman 8 weeks into the program. Overall, it seems that her weight is not changing, although it is fluctuating somewhat. (Printable graph paper can be downloaded from the Internet; see, e.g., *www. printablepaper.net/category/graph*).

Establishing Weekly Weighing: What to Do

Start weighing yourself once a week on a fixed morning of your choice. A weekday is usually best since on weekends you may dwell on any changes that have occurred. Do your best not to weigh yourself between these weekly weigh-ins.

Many people find this advice difficult to follow. On the one hand, if you are used to weighing yourself more often than weekly, you may feel uneasy reducing your frequency of weighing. You may be afraid that your weight will go up without you knowing. On the other hand, if you have been avoiding weighing yourself, you may be

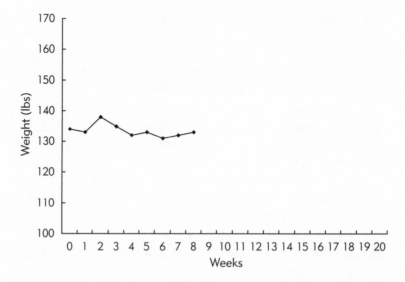

FIGURE 18. The weight graph of someone who is 8 weeks into the program.

afraid that restarting weighing will lead you to become preoccupied with your weight, and as a result you will want to weigh yourself more and more often. Whether or not either concern applies to you, do your best to weigh yourself once a week, and only once a week, on a preset day.

You may need to buy a scale. A normal domestic bathroom scale is perfectly adequate. Some people always weigh themselves when naked in an attempt to get as accurate a figure as possible. This is not necessary. As I stressed already, individual readings on the scale are difficult to interpret because of the influence of hydration and other factors including the state of one's bowels. Weighing yourself in light indoor clothing is absolutely fine.

If you are tempted to weigh yourself between your planned weekly weigh-ins, keep the scale out of sight and relatively inaccessible so that the temptation is easier to resist.

STEP 1 REVIEW SESSIONS

Your Step 1 review sessions should focus on the two elements of Step 1, monitoring and weekly weighing. You should hold the first review session after you have followed the Step 1 guidelines for 3 or 4 days and the next one after a further 3 or 4 days.

Each Step 1 review session should have two parts to it. The first is rereading Step 1 to remind yourself what you have been attempting to do, and the second is asking yourself the following four questions.

1. *Have I been monitoring?* If your answer is yes, you have made a good start. If your answer is no, there is a serious problem. Carefully consider your reasons for not monitoring, and perhaps reread the section on why monitoring is important. (It is a good idea, in fact, to reread the entire program at regular intervals. It is especially important to reread those sections on which you get stuck or make limited progress.)

Perhaps you should reconsider the advantages and disadvantages of deciding to change. If the advantages outweigh the disadvantages, you should make a fresh commitment to monitor as you are most unlikely to make significant progress without monitoring. Remember, monitoring provides you with important information and it helps you change.

2. *Can I improve my monitoring?* Study your monitoring records to see whether there is any room for improvement. Have you been following all the guidelines? For example, has your monitoring been accurate? Have you written everything you have eaten and drunk as soon as possible after their consumption? Have you bracketed meals? Have you used the asterisks in the way described? Have you been writing in column 6?

3. *Am I weighing myself once a week?* If so, well done! Record the number in column 6 of your records as well as on your summary sheet (described shortly). If you are weighing yourself more often than this, you should think why this is happening—you may need to put the scale out of sight or make it relatively inaccessible. If you are not weighing yourself at all, work out why. Remember you are embarking on this program in order to regain control over your eating, and your

weight may change as a result. It is much better to know what is happening than to keep your head in the sand and fear the worst.

4. *Are any patterns in my eating becoming evident?* Try to answer the following questions as carefully as possible. Doing so will increase your understanding of your binge eating problem and will highlight the things that need to be changed.

> Have I had any binges? Have they had anything in common? Have they happened at the same time of day? What about their triggers? Can I identify them?
>
> What have I eaten in my binges? Is there anything characteristic about the food? Why am I eating these particular foods? Are they foods I am avoiding at other times?
>
> What am I eating outside my binges? Am I attempting to limit my eating in any way? Am I delaying eating or avoiding eating? Am I eating normal meals?
>
> Are all my days the same, or do they differ? Are there days on which I diet and days when I binge?

Deciding When to Move on to Step 2

It is best not to move on to Step 2 immediately after your first review session. However, at the second review session (3 or 4 days later), you should ask yourself the same four questions:

> *Have I been monitoring?*
> *Can I improve my monitoring?*
> *Am I weighing myself once a week?*
> *Are any patterns becoming evident?*

Having done this, you are ready to make the first entry on your summary sheet. A blank sheet is shown in Figure 19 (which can also be found at my website). You will be using the summary sheet to chart your progress as you go through the program and to decide when to move on.

Guidelines for completing the summary sheet are given in Table 10. It should be filled in at the end of each week.

Week	B	V/L	CDs	Wt	Events
1					
2					
3					
4					
5					
6					
7					
8					
9					
10					
11					
12					
13					
14					
15					
16					
17					
18					
19					
20					

FIGURE 19. A blank summary sheet. An enlarged version of this fig-ure may be downloaded from *www.credo-oxford.com*.

Look at Figure 20, a partly completed summary sheet. It shows the progress of someone who is 6 weeks into the program. Now look at your own summary sheet. How many "change days" have you had? If you have had six or seven, you are ready to move on to Step 2. In that case, read through Step 2 and follow its advice while continuing with the two elements of Step 1, monitoring and weekly weighing. On the other hand, if you have had fewer than six or seven change days, try to work out why and continue with Step 1 until your next review session in a further 3 or 4 days' time. Then, once more, reexamine your progress and decide whether or not to move on.

Lastly, remember that it is important not to rush through the program. To get maximum benefit, you need to accomplish each step before moving on to the next.

TABLE 10. Instructions for completing the summary sheet.

Column 1: This indicates how many weeks you have been following the program. You have now completed your first week.

Column 2: Here record how many "binges" (B) you had over the last 7 days. You should obtain this figure from your monitoring records.

Column 3: This column is for recording the number of times you practiced any extreme method of weight control, such as self-induced vomiting or the misuse of laxatives or diuretics (V/L). Record each behavior separately. Again, you should get these figures from your monitoring records.

Column 4: Here record how many "change days" (CDs) you have had during the week. *A change day is one on which you did your best to follow the program.* Therefore at this point in the program *a change day is one on which you monitored accurately and you adhered to weekly weighing.* It does not matter whether or not you binged that day. The definition of a change day will alter as you work your way through the program.

Column 5: Record your weight (Wt) in this column. If you weighed yourself more than once during the week, record the weight on the day on which you had intended to weigh yourself.

Column 6: Here you should record other points of note. For example, note down when you move from one step of the program to the next. Also note any events that significantly influenced your eating; for example, being ill or away from home.

Week	B	V/L	CDs	Wt	Events
1	9		4	142	*Started Step 1*
2	7		7	144	*Off work this week*
3	4		5	143	*Step 2. Better week.*
4	1		7	139	*A good one! John here*
5	3		4	139	*Worse . . . need to try harder*
6	1		7	140	*Much better. Weekend with Julie*
7					
8					
9					
10					
11					
12					
13					
14					
15					
16					
17					
18					
19					
20					

FIGURE 20. A summary sheet completed by someone who is 6 weeks into the program.

STEP 2

Regular Eating

Step 1: Starting Well
Self-monitoring
Weekly weighing

Step 2: Regular Eating
Establishing a pattern of regular eating
Stopping vomiting and misusing laxatives or diuretics

Step 3: Alternatives to Binge Eating
Substituting alternative activities
Identifying changes in weight

Step 4: Problem Solving
Practicing problem solving

Step 5: Taking Stock
Reviewing progress
Deciding what else needs to be tackled

Dieting Module	Body Image Module
Tackling strict dieting	Addressing shape concerns, shape checking, shape avoidance, and feeling fat

Ending Well
Maintaining progress
Addressing setbacks

Establishing a pattern of regular eating is the single most significant change you can make when tackling a binge eating problem. One of the most consistent findings from over 30 years of research is that introducing a pattern of regular eating pushes aside most binges. Binge eating that was frequent becomes intermittent or stops altogether. To obtain this effect it is essential that you follow the guidelines below, so do read them carefully.

ESTABLISHING A PATTERN OF REGULAR EATING

You should aim to eat three planned meals each day, plus two or three planned snacks. Your eating pattern should therefore look something like this:

8:00 A.M.:   Breakfast
10:30 A.M.:   Midmorning snack
12:30 P.M.:   Lunch
3:30 P.M.:   Midafternoon snack
7:00 P.M.:   Evening meal
9:00 P.M.:   Evening snack

The exact times do not matter.

When introducing this eating pattern there are four main things to remember.

1. Plan ahead. At the beginning of each day (or the preceding evening), work out in advance when you are going to eat your meals and snacks, and write down the times at the top of the day's monitoring record. At all points in the day you should know when you are next going to have a meal or snack. If the day is going to be unpredictable, plan ahead as far as you can. Then, once you know what is next going to be happening, plan the remainder of the day.

2. Make sure you eat each of your planned meals and snacks. Do your best not to skip any of them.

3. It does not matter (at this stage) what you eat in the meals and snacks so long as you do not vomit or take laxatives or diuretics afterwards. Eat foods that you are comfortable with and, I shall shortly discuss, make sure you eat enough.

4. Do your utmost not to eat in the gaps between the meals and snacks. In this way your day will be divided up by the meals and snacks. They will be like stepping-stones through the day. So, morning will be the time between breakfast and lunch; early afternoon will be the period between lunch and your midafternoon snack; late afternoon will be between your midafternoon snack and your evening meal; and the evening will be divided in two by your evening snack. Breaking long periods of time into more manageable chunks of no longer than 3 to 4 hours contributes to the reduction in the frequency of binge eating. This is because many people are prone to binge when faced with extended periods of empty time.

Further Guidelines for Introducing "Regular Eating"

Your plan should be flexible rather than rigid. It is important that you adjust the times of your meals and snacks to suit your commitments, but do try to establish as regular a pattern as possible. Obviously, the precise times will vary from day to day; for instance, work days are likely to differ from nonwork ones.

When you eat should be dictated by your plan for the day and not by sensations of hunger or urges to eat. Popular articles in the media often tell us to listen to our body's signals and eat in response to them. This apparently wholesome advice ignores the fact that these signals are often disturbed in those who binge. Erratic eating, especially when it consists of alternating binge eating and dieting, disrupts the normal mechanisms that control hunger and fullness with the result that they are no longer a reliable guide as to when to eat. Later, once you have been eating regularly for some time, normal sensations of hunger and fullness will return—although this may take many months. Once this happens, you can use these sensations to guide your eating, although maintaining a pattern of regular eating should remain a priority.

Try not to leave more than 4 hours between the meals and snacks. Long gaps between episodes of eating create a mounting psychological and physiological pressure to eat that can eventually result in a binge. It is therefore wise to eat at regular intervals, with a 4-hour gap being the maximum. A possible exception to this "4-hour rule" is the morning because this is the time when most people are least likely to binge. If this applies to you, it would be reasonable to omit the midmorning snack as there are unlikely to be any negative effects.

Resist the temptation to compensate for the planned meals and snacks. There is no need to compensate for the planned meals and snacks, even if they are a new addition to your usual way of eating, as their introduction will reduce your frequency of binge eating, and therefore your calorie intake. Remember, this is true even if you vomit or take laxatives or diuretics immediately afterwards because none of these methods gets rid of anything like all the calories from the food that you have eaten. (If you have doubts about this statement, reread Chapters 4 and 5 to remind yourself about the ineffectiveness of these methods.)

> There is no need to compensate for the meals and snacks because their introduction reduces the frequency of binge eating, and therefore your calorie intake.

Some people are tempted to eat very little in their meals or snacks for fear of gaining weight. This is not wise since it will increase the risk of binge eating by creating physiological and psychological pressures to eat (as we discussed in Chapter 4). Introducing a pattern of regular eating has little, if any, effect on body weight.

What to eat. As noted above, it does not matter exactly what you eat in your meals and snacks so long as you eat enough. If you would like guidance on what to eat, the best advice is to consume a broad range of foods and average-sized portions. The size of an average portion can be determined from the eating habits of friends and relatives, from recipes, and from the labels on packaged meals. If someone is helping you follow the program, you might want to ask his or her advice on what is a reasonable amount to eat. The critical point is that it does not matter what you eat so long as you do not vomit or take laxatives or diuretics afterwards to compensate and so long as you eat enough.

Initially, this pattern of eating may create feelings of fullness. This is particularly likely if you are not used to eating without vomiting or taking laxatives or diuretics. The feelings of fullness almost invariably subside within an hour or so, and moreover, within a few weeks you will be less prone to have them. They are best dealt with by avoiding wearing tight clothes at mealtimes and by engaging in distracting activities for an hour or two afterwards (along the lines outlined in Step 3, p. 160).

Your planned pattern of eating should take priority over other activities. Do your best not to let other commitments take priority over your planned meals and snacks. At times, of course, your plan will need to be adjusted to accommodate important engagements. For example, if you know that your evening meal will have to be late, say at 10:00 P.M., then a sensible plan would be to move the evening snack earlier to midway between the midafternoon snack and the 10:00 P.M. evening meal.

If things go wrong, try to get back on track immediately. It is especially important to avoid writing off the remainder of a day because there was a problem earlier on. This "all-or-nothing" way of responding just makes matters worse. Always try to get back on track as soon as you can.

If your eating is very chaotic, you may not be able to introduce this eating pattern in one go. If this description applies to you, introduce the pattern in steps, starting with the part of the day that is least chaotic, which is usually the morning. So, begin by introducing breakfast and lunch (and possibly a midmorning snack) according to the guidelines above. Then, over the next few weeks, progressively introduce the other meals and snacks until the full pattern is in place.

Figure 21 shows a monitoring record completed by someone with bulimia nervosa who was at this stage in the program. You can see that at the top of the record she wrote when she planned to eat and that she did well at sticking to her plan.

Day *Thursday*   Date *July 23rd*

Time	Food and drink consumed	Place	*	V/L	Context and comments
	<u>Plan</u> Breakfast – 8 Lunch – 12:30 Aft snack – 3:30 Dinner – 7 Eve snack – 9				
7:40	Orange juice	Bedroom			Not sure about this
8:10	Bowl Bran Flakes Small bran muffin Decaf	Kitchen			Mustn't eat too much as I'm late and worried about work
10:45	Decaf	Office			
12.35	Turkey sandwich Potato salad (small) Apple Decaf 2 glasses of water	Staff room			Potato salad risky. Lunch a bit too large but it was planned
3:15	Apple Diet coke	Office			
7:00	Large slice pepperoni pizza Vanilla ice cream—2 scoops Decaf	Kitchen	*		Ice cream not planned ... bad!
9:30	Small slice apple pie	Kitchen			Back on track

FIGURE 21. A monitoring record of someone 4 weeks into the program.

Introducing Regular Eating: What to Do

Introduce this pattern of eating while continuing to monitor. Do not expect this to be easy. You may well have problems. For example, you are likely to want to eat when you should not; conversely, you might not want to eat when you should, especially after you have binged. Do your very best, while at the same time noting down on your monitoring records any difficulties you are having. The suggestions made below regarding meals, shopping, and cooking may help you deal with some of these difficulties. Further suggestions are made in Steps 3 and 4.

So, start eating this way and assess your progress at the end of each day. Then make whatever adjustments seem appropriate. For example, you may discover that you are having your evening snack so late in the day that it is not breaking up the evening. In that case, try moving it to an earlier time.

Remember also to complete your summary sheet at the end of each week. A "change day" at this stage is one on which you monitored accurately, weighed weekly, and did your best to stick to your planned pattern of eating, irrespective of whether you binged.

WHAT TO DO
ABOUT SELF-INDUCED VOMITING

If you make yourself vomit after binge eating, and only then, your vomiting will go away as you introduce the pattern of regular eating. This is because it is tied to your binge eating (see Chapter 4, p. 49)— it will resolve as your binge eating resolves.

For the first few weeks you may experience a strong urge to vomit after some of the planned meals or snacks. If this is the case, you should do your best to distract yourself until the urge has declined (usually within an hour or so). You might also want to make vomiting more difficult by staying in the company of others.

If you are someone who vomits at times other than after binge eating, and you are unable to break this habit, you should seek professional help. This way of eating can be difficult to overcome on your own.

WHAT TO DO ABOUT LAXATIVE AND DIURETIC MISUSE

As we discussed in Chapter 4, some people with binge eating problems misuse laxatives or diuretics. This misuse takes two forms. They may take them to compensate for specific episodes of overeating, in which case the behavior is very similar to self-induced vomiting. Alternatively, they may take them on a more routine basis, independent of particular episodes of overeating, in which case the behavior is more like dieting.

What has just been said about self-induced vomiting applies equally to the first type of laxative misuse. It will cease as binge eating ceases. However, if you have been taking laxatives or diuretics independently of binge eating, my advice is to make a firm decision to stop taking them from now on. Most people are capable of doing this, especially once they know how ineffective these drugs are at preventing calorie absorption (see p. 76).

If you have been taking laxatives or diuretics on an occasional basis then you can stop taking them in one go. However, as you may recall from Chapter 5 (p. 77), if you have been taking them on most days, stopping suddenly can result in a period of fluid retention lasting a week or so, and obviously this will result in weight gain. It is therefore better to phase the drugs out, perhaps by halving your daily intake each week. In the unlikely event that you experience fluid retention (evidence of which is swelling of the hands and feet), it is important to keep in mind that the accompanying weight gain is accounted for by water, not fat, and that it is temporary. It will go away within a few weeks as the excess water is lost. Nevertheless, you should see your physician if you experience fluid retention as it is potentially serious and it can have other causes.

SOME ADVICE ON EATING IN
AND EATING OUT

People with binge eating problems often find mealtimes difficult, especially when eating out. Below are some useful tips, although some of the suggestions may not be relevant to you. I suggest that you read through them and try those that apply. *Keep in mind that you will not have to behave this way forever.* These are interim measures designed to help you regain control over your eating. You will be able to drop them once they are no longer relevant.

Restrict your eating to certain places in your home. Part of regaining control over eating involves formalizing your eating habits. When you eat at home it is a good idea to have one or two set places where you eat. These should be at a table or its equivalent, and not within an arm's reach of supplies of food. You should not eat in your bedroom or in the bathroom. If you have only one room, it is best to restrict your eating to one place in the room.

When eating, concentrate on what you are doing. While it may be tempting to distract yourself when eating, this is not a good idea. Instead, focus on what you are doing. Try to savor your food. You also need to ensure that you are not eating in an abnormal way. For example, check to see that you are not eating too fast. Being aware of what you are doing will also help to reduce the chance that your meals and snacks evolve into binges. For this reason try not to engage in other activities (such as watching television) when eating. Also, sit down, as eating on the move can result in inadvertent "grazing."

When eating, restrict the availability of food. When eating a meal or snack, have only the preplanned amount of food at hand. Whenever practicable, keep packages and serving dishes off the table in case you are tempted to eat more than you had intended.

If need be, impose some controls over the way you are eating. If you tend to eat automatically or rapidly, practice putting down your utensils between mouthfuls and insert pauses into your meals. Also practice leaving food on the plate. This may seem wasteful, but anything that will minimize the likelihood of binge eating is not truly wasteful. And discard leftovers because at this stage in the program they may be too tempting to resist.

When eating with others, do not be persuaded to eat more than you had planned. It is not uncommon to be put under pressure to have second helpings or larger quantities than you want. You must resist this pressure. Practice polite but firm ways of declining—for example, "No, thank you. I really have had enough. It was delicious." If someone still puts unwanted food on your plate, leave it untouched. Under such circumstances it is the other person who is being impolite, not you.

When eating a meal out, take stock between courses. It is easy for meals in restaurants or at other people's homes to get out of hand. You may not know how many courses there will be or what they will contain. You therefore need to keep a careful eye on what is happening and take stock at intervals. Make some excuse—for example, that you have to make a quick phone call—so that you can leave the table and collect your thoughts. Ideally, get out your recording sheet and complete it while thinking over what to do next. In meals with a large number of courses, it is often easier to skip one or two courses altogether than to try to limit the amount you eat at each one.

Buffets are a particular challenge. The best approach is to take some time to look over what is being offered, and then step away to give yourself some moments to plan exactly what you are going to eat. Once you have finished eating, get rid of your plate and utensils and stay well away from the food.

Although you may not feel like doing this, it is a good idea not to drink too much alcohol when eating out as otherwise your judgment and willpower will be impaired.

SOME ADVICE ON SHOPPING AND COOKING

Many people with binge eating problems also have difficulties with shopping and cooking. Here are some tips for addressing these difficulties. Remember, as with the advice concerning mealtimes, not all the suggestions may be relevant to you.

Limit your stock of foods on which you are likely to binge. At this stage in the program it is best to restrict your access to foods that either trigger your binges or comprise them. It is unhelpful having them around. Therefore, when shopping, avoid buying these foods. If this is not practicable, limit the quantities that you purchase.

Ensure that you have adequate supplies of foods that are acceptable to you. It is important that you have a ready supply of food that you feel comfortable eating.

Plan your shopping. For the meantime do not shop for food on the spur of the moment. Instead, plan your shopping in advance and adhere to your shopping list. If possible, avoid shopping when hungry and on days when you feel at risk of binge eating. Shopping online can be helpful.

When cooking, avoid tasting the food. Picking at what you are cooking can trigger binges. Some people find it helpful to chew gum since this makes picking almost impossible.

Avoid unnecessary exposure to food. As we discussed in Chapter 4, many people with binge eating problems are preoccupied with thoughts about food and eating, and this can fuel an interest in food and cooking. Partly as a result, some spend a lot of time cooking for others. This should be resisted since, for obvious reasons, unnecessary exposure to food is risky. Some have a tendency to press food on others. This is not a good idea. Instead, treat others as you would want to be treated yourself. Offer food, but do not put people under pressure to eat more than they want. It is also not uncommon for people with binge eating problems to work directly or indirectly with food. If this applies to you and you can see that it is contributing to your eating problem, you should seriously consider changing your job.

STEP 2 REVIEW SESSIONS

It usually takes a few weeks to establish a pattern of regular eating. It may take longer. You should review your progress twice a week. On each occasion study your monitoring records, and once a week complete the summary sheet. A "change day" at this point is one on which you monitored accurately; you adhered to weekly weighing; and you did your best to stick to a planned pattern of regular eating, whether or not you binged.

Each Step 2 review session should have three parts to it. The first is rereading Step 2 to remind yourself what you have been trying to do. The second part is asking yourself the four questions from Step 1:

Have I been monitoring?
Can I improve my monitoring?
Are any patterns in my eating becoming evident?
Am I weighing myself once a week?

The third part is asking yourself the following eight questions regarding Step 2.

1. *Each day, am I planning regular meals and snacks?* Remember, to get control over your eating, you need to stay one step ahead of the problem, rather than be one step behind it. Each morning (or the previous evening if this suits you better) you should work out when you will be eating the next day's meals and snacks, and you should do your best to stick to this plan. This way you will be more likely to foresee problems than come upon them unawares.

2. *Am I trying to restrict my eating to the day's meals and snacks?* This is also central to the program.

3. *Am I skipping any of the meals and snacks?* It is important that you do not skip any meals or snacks as doing so will make you vulnerable to binge.

4. *Are the gaps between my meals and snacks longer than 4 hours?* For the same reason, the gaps between your meals and snacks should not be long, and never longer than 4 hours.

5. *Am I eating between my meals and snacks?* The goal is to restrict your eating to the planned meals and snacks. If you are succeeding in doing this, your monitoring records will have a clear pattern to them. Furthermore, this pattern should match the plan written at the top.

6. *Am I getting back on track when things go wrong?* It is important not to give up whenever something goes wrong. There is a tendency

for people with binge eating problems to view days as a single unit with the result that when anything goes wrong they see the whole day as being ruined. This is not helpful and is an example of all-or-nothing thinking.

When you start to introduce a pattern of regular eating you will still be having binges. Do not feel despondent about this. The important thing is that after each binge you get back on track as soon as possible rather than delay until the next day. Try hard not to skip the next meal or snack because this will only make you vulnerable to binge again.

7. *Am I adjusting the timing of my meals and snacks to accommodate events and circumstances?* Your eating pattern must not be too rigid—otherwise you will run into difficulties when faced with special occasions. Examine your monitoring records to see whether there have been any such times and review how well you have dealt with them.

8. *Am I following the advice regarding vomiting and the misuse of laxatives and diuretics?* As we discussed in Chapter 4, all these behaviors encourage binge eating. It is therefore essential that you stop them by following the advice in this chapter.

Deciding When to Move on to Step 3

Most people need to spend quite a few weeks consolidating this way of eating. However, you do not need to wait until you have established a pattern of regular eating before moving on. This is because Step 3 will help you follow Step 2. What is essential is that you are having six or seven change days each week. If you are not, then you should reread Step 2 and stay at this stage for at least another week.

Step 3 will help you follow Step 2.

If you are ready to move on, continue with Steps 1 and 2 while starting to implement Step 3.

STEP 3

Alternatives to Binge Eating

Step 1: Starting Well
Self-monitoring
Weekly weighing

Step 2: Regular Eating
Establishing a pattern of regular eating
Stopping vomiting and misusing laxatives or diuretics

Step 3: Alternatives to Binge Eating
Substituting alternative activities
Identifying changes in weight

Step 4: Problem Solving
Practicing problem solving

Step 5: Taking Stock
Reviewing progress
Deciding what else needs to be tackled

Dieting Module
Tackling strict
dieting

Body Image Module
Addressing shape concerns, shape
checking, shape avoidance, and feeling fat

Ending Well
Maintaining progress
Addressing setbacks

In essence, there are two aspects to establishing a pattern of "regular eating." One is introducing the planned meals and snacks, and the other is not eating in the gaps between them. Step 3 is designed to help you not eat in the gaps. It also provides advice on how to tell whether your weight is changing or not.

When starting to adopt a pattern of regular eating, it is common for there to be urges to eat between the meals and snacks, and perhaps urges to vomit following them. It is a common mistake to assume that these urges will mount and mount until they become impossible to resist. In reality, they will rise to a peak and then gradually decline. The challenge is not to give in to them for the hour or so when they are at their worst which is best done by actively distracting yourself. How to do this depends upon the circumstances, but it is useful to have prepared in advance a list of things you might do.

PREPARING TO USE
ALTERNATIVE ACTIVITIES

The first step is to think of activities that might help you resist urges to eat or vomit. These will be needed for the hour or so when the urges are at their most intense. People's choices of activities differ, but here are some typical ones:

> Going for a brisk walk or bicycle ride
> Telephoning or visiting friends or relatives
> Exercising
> E-mailing
> Going on Facebook
> Browsing the Internet
> Playing a video game
> Taking a bath or shower
> Watching an engaging movie or a favorite television program

The goal is that you create a list of activities that suits you personally. In general, each activity needs to have three properties:

1. It is active (i.e., it involves doing something) rather than passive (such as watching whatever happens to be on television).
2. It is enjoyable (i.e., it doesn't feel like a chore).
3. It is realistic (i.e., it is something that you are likely to do).

Here is another useful tip. Go through your music collection and identify pieces of music that you enjoy and are mood-enhancing. You may well find that music is good at changing your frame of mind and thereby at helping you deal with urges to eat or vomit. Keep such music at hand, ready for use at difficult times. Indeed, you might like to create a specific playlist for this purpose.

Once you have constructed your list of activities, write them down on a card or keep an e-note of them somewhere handy. Your list needs to be readily accessed whenever you have urges to eat or vomit.

You also need to get expert at identifying these urges. It is important to spot them early when they are easier to deal with. So, as soon as you detect an urge of this type, note it down in column 6 of your monitoring record and get out your list of alternative activities.

SUBSTITUTING ALTERNATIVE ACTIVITIES

Say it is 7:00 P.M., and you have eaten your evening meal. Perhaps you feel that you ate too much and you are tempted to vomit or to give up and binge. Perhaps you are also tired, having had a stressful day, and you have nothing planned for the evening. Clearly you are at risk. Now, if you are recording properly, you will be well aware that a potential problem is looming. You will be one step ahead of the problem. You will have written down your evening meal and also something in column 6 along the following lines: "Feel as if I've eaten too much. I'm tired, and there's a long evening ahead of me. Strong urge to binge." What should you do under such circumstances?

There are two related problems here. The first is your urge to vomit or binge, and the second is the fact that you have nothing to do. This step of the program, Step 3, addresses the first of these problems, the urge to vomit or binge. Step 4 is concerned with addressing day-to-day difficulties such as having nothing to do.

Returning to the urge to vomit or binge, two things need to happen:

1. Time must pass. These urges fade with time. Even half an hour may be long enough for the urge to decline sufficiently for you to be able to resist it easily.
2. You need to engage in something distracting—something that is active, enjoyable, and realistic.

So, you need to get out your list of activities and review it. It is 7:00 P.M., and you have no plans for the evening. What could you do? You decide to do two things. First, you decide to exercise since, although you don't feel in the mood, you know that you will feel better for having done so, and you will not be tempted to eat while exercising. Also, exercising will help you unwind. But, before starting to exercise, you also decide to call some friends to see if it is possible to meet up later on. And all the time you are aware that you are going to have an evening snack at around 9:00 P.M.

With a plan like this it is likely that you will resist the urge to eat. Contacting friends will be distracting and, with any luck, will give you something positive to look forward to. Exercising and then taking a shower will occupy time and will make you feel better about yourself.

Plans like this work. At first, you may find that urges to eat or vomit take quite a while to subside. However, they will fade more and more quickly with practice. Eventually the urges will disappear altogether or become so weak that you can ignore them.

"Urge surfing," as this process is sometimes called, can have one adverse effect. This is that you may become aware of unpleasant thoughts and feelings that were previously obscured by binge eating. In reality, this is a positive development because it enables you to address them directly rather than sweep them under the carpet. Step 4 discusses how to do this.

Substituting Alternative Activities: What to Do

You need to practice engaging in alternative activities when you experience urges to eat or vomit. Assess your progress at each of your review sessions. Also, remember to complete your summary sheet each week. Classify as a "change day" any day on which you monitored accurately; you adhered to weekly weighing; you did your best to stick to your planned pattern of regular eating, as described in Step 2, whether or not you also binged; and you used your list of alternative activities to deal with urges to eat or vomit.

STEP 3 REVIEW SESSIONS

At each review session you should study your monitoring records and summary sheet (completed weekly) and ask yourself the four questions below, in addition to those relating to Steps 1 and 2.

1. *Have I devised a list of alternative activities?* You should have created a list and be carrying it with you. If you are to intervene when you need to, you will need this list at hand. The list may well require amendment on the basis of experience: some activities may work; others may not.

2. *Am I recording urges to eat or vomit?* You should be recording these urges in column 6 of your monitoring records. If you are to intervene successfully, you must record these urges at the time that you experience them rather than some time afterwards.

Look through the monitoring records that you have completed since starting Step 3. Have there been urges to eat or vomit? Did you record them when they occurred? If you have been eating at times other than your planned meals and snacks, this suggests that you have had such urges.

3. *Am I using my list of alternative activities when needed?* If you have had an urge to eat between your meals and snacks, or to vomit, have you used your list of activities?

4. Could my use of alternative activities be improved? If you have attempted to intervene, how did it go? Did you intervene early enough? Did you engage in one or more of the activities on your list? Which activities worked, and which did not? Have you modified your list accordingly?

It is best to have a review session like this at least once or twice a week.

Deciding When to Move On to Step 4

It is impossible to specify how long you should spend on this step since you may or may not be having opportunities to practice using alternative activities. Certainly, if your review sessions indicate that you are having urges to eat or vomit, but you are not successfully addressing them, you should delay moving on. As stressed already, the successful use of alternative activities requires practice. It is important that you take every opportunity to do so.

WHAT IS HAPPENING TO MY WEIGHT?

By this point in the program it should be becoming clear what is happening to your weight. Most people find that there has been little or no change, although there may well have been fluctuations. As we discussed earlier (p. 139), if you want to be scientific about this matter, plot your weekly weights on a graph. An example is shown in Figure 22. But before you do this, it is important to note that inter-preting weight graphs is more difficult than many people realize. This is for three main reasons:

1. Each weight has a degree of uncertainty around it, mainly due to variation in the body's state of hydration. It is impossible to know how hydrated you are when you weigh yourself, yet this has a big influence on your weight and how it changes from day to day (as I discussed in Chapter 5, p. 66).

2. Until quite a few weeks have passed, it is more or less impossible to work out whether your weight is increasing, is decreasing, or is stable because there is insufficient information to reveal the emerging trend.

3. To work out what is happening to your weight, you need to focus on the past 4 or more weeks, rather than on the latest number on the scale. This is because individual readings are almost impossible to interpret due to the uncertainty that surrounds each one of them.

> *You need to focus on the past 4 or more weeks, rather than on the latest number on the scale.*

With these points in mind, look at your weight graph and see if you can identify what is happening to your weight. If you have one, use a transparent ruler to identify the emerging trend. Figure 23 shows a weight graph in which the dotted straight line highlights the underlying trend (i.e., the line represents where the ruler would

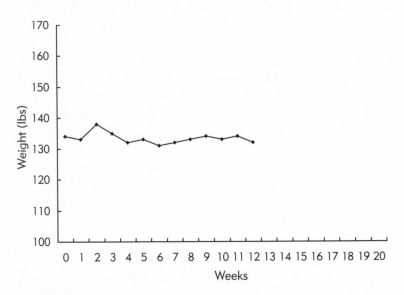

FIGURE 22. The weight graph of someone 12 weeks into the program.

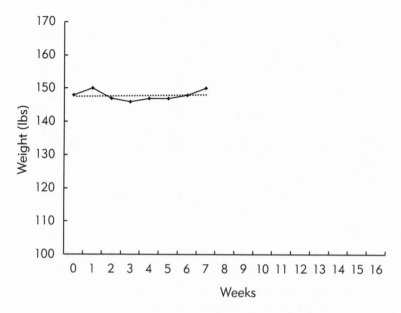

FIGURE 23. The weight graph of someone 7 weeks into the program. The dotted line highlights the underlying trend.

be placed). Note that the line does not intersect with the latest reading—this is often the case. Two tips are worth noting in this context. First, turning the weight graph 90 degrees and looking at it vertically can highlight a trend that was not apparent when the graph was inspected from the usual horizontal viewpoint. Second, if you are struggling to be objective, imagine the graph is of something of less personal significance (say, weekly rainfall over the past month).

At this stage in the program, it is likely that you will conclude that there has been little or no change in your weight. However, we need to consider two possibilities.

1. *Your weight has fallen consistently since starting the program, and you are now underweight* (see Table 8, p. 125). If this is the case, you should see your physician, explain what you have been doing, and get advice. The program may not be suitable for you. It is

possible that you are eating too little during your meals and snacks. This is a potential problem since it will limit your ability to stop binge eating.

2. Your weight has risen consistently while following the program. If this applies, you need to check two things. The first is whether you are now "overweight," medically speaking (see Appendix II, p. 216). If this is the case, you might want to discuss this problem with your physician. If you decide

Appendix III discusses what to do if you have a binge eating problem and are overweight.

to do this, you should explain that you are following a scientifically tested program that is designed to help you regain control over your eating. It is not a weight loss program. Appendix III discusses what to do if you have a binge eating problem and are overweight. As we noted earlier (p. 121), you will be in a much better position to control your weight once you have control over your eating.

The second matter to consider is whether you were somewhat underweight when you started the program. If so, it is not unlikely that your weight is now increasing to a more healthy level. This is a good thing, although you may be finding it difficult to accept.

What you must not do is go on a strict diet because this would be likely to undo any progress you have made so far.

STEP 4

Problem Solving

Step 1: Starting Well
Self-monitoring
Weekly weighing

Step 2: Regular Eating
Establishing a pattern of regular eating
Stopping vomiting and misusing laxatives or diuretics

Step 3: Alternatives to Binge Eating
Substituting alternative activities
Identifying changes in weight

Step 4: Problem Solving
Practicing problem solving

Step 5: Taking Stock
Reviewing progress
Deciding what else needs to be tackled

Dieting Module	Body Image Module
Tackling strict dieting	Addressing shape concerns, shape checking, shape avoidance, and feeling fat

Ending Well
Maintaining progress
Addressing setbacks

Most binges do not occur at random. As I described in Chapter 1, many are triggered by unpleasant events or circumstances including problems with relationships. It is therefore important to develop your skills for tackling problems of this type. This is the focus of Step 4. And even if your binges are not generally triggered by external forces, most people find that developing their problem-solving skills is of value to them.

DEVELOPING YOUR
PROBLEM-SOLVING SKILLS

How people solve problems has been extensively studied, as has how to help people become better at it. What follows are guidelines for becoming a good problem solver.

How to Solve Problems

Efficient problem solving involves six steps. Good problem solvers go through these steps without being aware of it. You can become a good problem solver too by following the same process. In an informal way you have already been doing something like this when addressing your urges to binge in Step 3. Now it is time to formalize the process.

Effective problem solving involves the following six steps:

Step 1: Identifying the problem as early as possible.
Step 2: Specifying the problem accurately.
Step 3: Considering as many solutions as possible.
Step 4: Thinking through the implications of each solution.
Step 5: Choosing the best solution or combination of solutions.
Step 6: Acting on the solution.

If you are trying to enhance your problem solving, there is a seventh step. This involves looking back over how well you have "problem-solved." We will now discuss each of these steps in some detail.

Step 1: Identifying the Problem as Early as Possible. Spotting problems early can prevent them from becoming overwhelming. In the example we considered in Step 3 (p. 161), you could have spotted the problem—having nothing planned for the evening—during the afternoon if you had been thinking ahead. Next best would have been spotting the problem as soon as it arose, say on finishing your evening meal.

There may be clues that a problem is developing. Maybe you are feeling fed up or beginning to have an urge to binge. Urges to binge are often a sure sign that there is a problem afoot, so whenever you have such an urge you should consider whether there is a problem lurking behind it.

Sometimes you will find that there is more than one problem. When this is the case, distinguish the two and problem-solve them separately because their solutions may differ.

Step 2: Specifying the Problem Accurately. Working out the true nature of the problem is essential if you are to find the right solution. If we return to the same example, you might have thought that the problem was the urge to binge. In fact the urge was your reaction to the true problem, which was that you had nothing to do all evening and you were tired. So, properly specified, the problem was "I have nothing to do this evening and I am tired."

Step 3: Considering as Many Solutions as Possible. Do not censor yourself. Be creative. Try to think of all possible solutions. This way you are more likely to come up with a good one. Returning to our example, you might come up with these possible solutions:

Watch television.
Go to bed.
Go on Facebook.
Call some friends to see if they are free.
Clean the apartment.
Go for a jog.

Step 4: Thinking Through the Implications of Each Solution.
Staying with our example, here are the likely ramifications of each of the above solutions:

> *Watch television.* This is not a great idea since there is nothing worth watching and I will therefore get bored. This will make the risk of binge eating even greater.
>
> *Go to bed.* This is also not a good idea. It is how I react when I am fed up, and it solves nothing. Indeed, it makes me feel worse. What tends to happen is that it makes me feel even sorrier for myself. It makes me feel like a failure, and eventually I get up and binge.
>
> *Go on Facebook.* This is probably a bad idea right now. I am not feeling good about myself, and seeing what everyone else is doing might well make me feel worse.
>
> *Call some friends.* This is not a bad idea. When I feel this way I usually hide away, but if someone calls it often cheers me up, especially if we can arrange to meet. Why should I wait for them to call me? I could just as well call them. If they are busy, they can always say so.
>
> *Clean the apartment.* It's clean enough already! I need to get a life! I don't have to be productive all the time.
>
> *Go for a jog.* This is not a bad idea in principle, but given my present weight I don't enjoy jogging. Also, I have eaten too much, and it's raining. I suppose I could go for a brisk walk. This would serve the same function since it would help me let off steam while I would also feel good about having exercised. And what's so bad about getting wet!

Step 5: Choosing the Best Solution or Combination of Solutions. Choosing the best solution is often not difficult. If you have come up with a good number of potential solutions and carefully thought through their implications, the best solution or combination of solutions is usually fairly clear.

Returning to the example, you decide that calling some friends and exercising are the best options. Note that these are also the alternative activities that you chose to help cope with the urge to eat (in Step 3 of the program). When this happens, they are likely to be especially effective.

Step 6: Acting on the Solution. The final step is to put your solution(s) into practice. You do not have to stick rigidly to the chosen solution, if it turns out not to be a good idea, try one of the other solutions.

The Extra Step: Reviewing Your Problem Solving. To become an efficient problem solver, you need to take one crucial final step. This involves *reviewing the entire problem-solving process, usually the next day, to see whether you could have done it any better.* The matter at hand is not whether you solved the problem in question, although this is relevant, but rather it is how well you problem-solved. Maybe you overcame the problem but did not problem-solve very well (e.g., you thought of just one possible solution and simply got on with it). While this was a success in one sense, it wasn't a success in terms of becoming a good problem solver. It is important to remember that the goal is that you become a good problem solver. You are trying to develop a skill.

Returning to our example, say you first called three friends. Two of them were in. Neither was free to meet there and then, but you caught up with each other's news and made arrangements to meet in the next week or so. You then forced yourself to go out for a long fast walk. You were out for nearly 40 minutes. This made you feel tired (and you got soaked), but you felt healthier and happier when you got home, and the urge to binge had passed. By this time it was 9:15 P.M. and time for your planned evening snack.

The next day you reviewed your problem solving. You considered each step one by one. You thought that you could have done better at identifying the problem early. Looking back, you saw that it would have been perfectly possible to have spotted it in the afternoon, before you left work. On the other hand, you accomplished the other five steps pretty well. It certainly demonstrated that you could address such circumstances, whereas in the past you would have had a binge and felt even worse.

Developing Your Problem-Solving Skills

Practice problem solving as often as possible. You can practice it on more or less any type of problem. It can be used to address problems entirely separate from the eat-

> *Problem solving can be used to address more or less any type of problem, including problems at work or in your relationships.*

ing problem, such as problems at work or in your relationships.

Do note that when problem solving, it is far better to write out each step than it is to prob-

lem-solve in your head. From now on, look out for problems, and each time you identify one, work through the six steps and then review the entire process the following day.

It is a good idea to use your monitoring records for this purpose. Write "Problem" in column 6 and then turn the sheet over and work through the six steps on the back. Also write down the findings of your review (the extra step). Figures 24 and 25 show monitoring records that illustrate the example that we have just discussed.

Proactive Problem Solving

A recent refinement of this process is called "proactive problem solving." It is designed for people who tend to be rather late in identifying problems. It is generally the case that problems spotted early are easier to address than those spotted later on. So, if this applies to you, become a proactive problem solver by repeatedly screening the rest of your day for possible problems. A simple way of doing this is to screen the remainder of the day every time you make an entry on your monitoring records. In this way you keep looking out for potential difficulties and problem-solve them then and there.

Day _Monday_   Date _Nov 3rd_

Time	Food and drink consumed	Place	*	V/L	Context and comments
	Plan Breakfast – 8 Lunch – 12:30 Aft snack – 3 Dinner – 6:30 Eve snack – 9:30				
8:40	Coffee Bowl granola }	Kitchen			
10:45	Coffee	Work			Very busy at work – too much to do. Unrealistic deadline.
12:40	Tomato soup Slice bread Large orange Coffee }	Work			Quick lunch
3:15	2 Oreos	Office	*		Tired ... shouldn't have had the second one.
6:45	Lasagne-large slice Salad and Italian dressing Diet Coke }	Kitchen			Left over from yesterday. Ate it too fast and without thinking. Really stressed. Nothing to do this evening. Strong urge to binge. PROBLEM
9:15	Bowl fruit salad	Kitchen			Survived without bingeing! → Going to have an early night

FIGURE 24. A monitoring record showing a "problem."

1. Done.

2. I have nothing to do all evening and I am tired and stressed after a bad day at work.

3. — TV   — Call friends
   — Go to bed   — Clean apartment
   — Facebook   — Jog

4. TV—nothing I want to watch, risky
   Go to bed—terrible idea; will end up feeling even worse
   Facebook— likely to be annoying
   Call friends—good idea; not done this for ages
   Clean apartment— it is clean enough!
   Jog—eaten too much; don't feel like it, raining

5. Call friends. If that doesn't work, go for a fast walk

REVIEW (NEXT DAY)

Could have spotted the problem in the afternoon—would have given me more options.

Otherwise did well. Spoke to K who I've not spoken to for ages. Great to catch up. Going to see each other next weekend. Felt much better after the call. Didn't need to go for the walk.

AVOIDED A CERTAIN BINGE!

FIGURE 25. The back of the monitoring record shown in Figure 24 showing a successful attempt at problem solving.

STEP 4 REVIEW SESSIONS

At each review session you should study your monitoring records and summary sheet and ask yourself the three questions below, in addition to those relating to Steps 1, 2, and 3.

1. *Am I problem solving frequently enough?* It is important to look out for opportunities to practice your problem-solving skills, whether or not the problem might lead to a binge. Any problem, however trivial, will provide you with a chance to develop your skills.

You might feel that problem solving is "obsessive" and not your style. Be that as it may, it is worth the effort and will not have to be continued forever. Many people are surprised at how useful they find the technique. Some continue with it long after their eating problem has gone. Others abandon it once it no longer seems relevant. For now, it is important to practice problem solving.

2. *When I am problem solving, am I doing it properly?* It is important that you follow the six steps and write them down at the time. This will help you think clearly and it will also assist the review process afterwards.

3. *Am I reviewing my problem solving?* Reviewing each attempt at problem solving is central to developing your problem-solving skills. Remember, the matter at hand is not whether the problem was solved (although hopefully it was) but rather whether you followed the six steps as well as you could. Could your problem solving have been any better?

Also, remember to complete your summary sheet each week. Classify as a "change day" any day on which you monitored accurately; you adhered to weekly weighing; you did your best to stick to your planned pattern of eating, as described in Step 2, whether or not you also binged; you used your list of alternative activities to deal with any urges to eat or vomit, as described in Step 3; and you practiced problem solving at every available opportunity, as described here.

Deciding When to Move On to Step 5

As before, it is not possible to provide specific guidelines for when to move on as you may or may not be having opportunities to problem-solve. This said, if your binge eating is becoming infrequent, or you have been at Steps 2, 3, and 4 for 6 to 8 weeks, now is a good time to move on to Step 5 and take stock.

STEP 5

Taking Stock

Step 1: Starting Well
Self-monitoring
Weekly weighing

Step 2: Regular Eating
Establishing a pattern of regular eating
Stopping vomiting and misusing laxatives or diuretics

Step 3: Alternatives to Binge Eating
Substituting alternative activities
Identifying changes in weight

Step 4: Problem Solving
Practicing problem solving

Step 5: Taking Stock
Reviewing progress
Deciding what else needs to be tackled

Dieting Module	**Body Image Module**
Tackling strict dieting	Addressing shape concerns, shape checking, shape avoidance, and feeling fat

Ending Well
Maintaining progress
Addressing setbacks

If you are binge eating intermittently, or you have been at Steps 2, 3, and 4 for 6 to 8 weeks, it is a good time to take stock. By "taking stock," I mean reviewing in detail how you are getting on. To do this, you will need your summary sheet.

SHOULD I CONTINUE WITH THE PROGRAM?

By now, if the program is going to help you, you should be seeing definite signs that you are benefiting. Introducing a pattern of regular eating (Step 2) should have had the effect of displacing many of your binges, and engaging in alternative activities should have helped you resist urges to binge (Step 3). And problem solving (Step 4) should be helping you deal with the type of day-to-day difficulties that tend to trigger your binges. But things may not be improving or you may feel that the program is not for you. This is a good time to take stock. See which of the following "outcomes" applies to you.

1. *Things are going well.* If the frequency of your binges has clearly decreased (and, if applicable, so has your vomiting and/or use of laxatives or diuretics), you should continue with the program. These are very promising signs, and you are doing well.

2. *There has been little change, but you have not been following the program as well as you could.* If you are not benefiting in terms of your eating, but you know that you are not following the program as well as you could, you need to question your commitment to change. Reread the section "Why Change?" at the beginning of Part II (p. 119) to remind yourself why you embarked upon the program. If you conclude that you really do want to change, you should consider restarting, perhaps after a short break. On the other hand, if you are unsure whether you want to change—perhaps it all seems too much effort, or this is the wrong time—then it might be better to stop. You can always restart at some point in the future.

3. *There has been little change despite your best efforts.* If you are doing your best to change, a good measure of which is the number of "change days" you are having each week, yet the frequency of your binges has not altered significantly, the program is not working. There are various reasons why this might be the case. The eating problem may simply be too severe to tackle by yourself or the processes maintaining the eating problem (described in Chapter 4) may be so powerful that any inroads you do make simply do not last. If either appears to be the case, you should seriously consider getting outside help. Guidance for doing so is provided in Appendix I.

Another possibility is that one or more associated problems are getting in the way of you making progress. It is not uncommon for people with eating problems to have other difficulties. These vary, the most common being a clinical depression; difficulties with self-esteem and assertiveness; problems with perfectionism; and unsatisfactory relationships and life circumstances. If these accompanying difficulties are not severe, they do not necessarily obstruct progress. And, indeed, overcoming the binge eating problem can have a positive effect on them—for example, overcoming an eating problem often results in an improvement in mood, self-esteem, and relationships. However, if these accompanying problems are marked they can be a barrier to change. Here are two

> *The most common accompanying difficulties are a clinical depression, low self-esteem, problems with assertiveness, and unsatisfactory relationships and life circumstances.*

> *Overcoming an eating problem often has a positive effect on accompanying problems such as depression, self-esteem, and relationship problems.*

examples. The day-to-day stress that arises from relationship problems can trigger episodes of binge eating and unless the relationship problem improves the binge eating may prove impossible to overcome. Alternatively, you may be prone to perfectionism. If so, you will have high standards. This is fine, but if your standards are so high that nothing is really good enough, this will interfere with your progress through the program.

If you have accompanying difficulties of this type and they are obstructing your progress, then they need to be addressed. To do so you have two options; either tackle the difficulty yourself or get pro-

fessional help. If you choose the former route, Appendix IV (Tackling
"Other Problems") provides guidance as to how to proceed. Which-
ever option you choose, you may

> *If you have a difficulty that is obstructing your progress, then this difficulty will need to be addressed.*

need to suspend the program for the meantime and instead focus
your efforts on overcoming the accompanying difficulty. The one

> *Often relationship problems can be successfully addressed using the problem-solving approach.*

exception can be relationship problems. Often they can be successfully
addressed using the problem-solving
approach that you learned in Step 4.

WHAT NEXT?

Assuming you are going to continue
with the program, now is the time to
plan its remaining steps. Exactly what
they should be depends upon the nature
of your binge eating problem and, more

> *To plan the remainder of the program, you will need to reread Chapter 4.*

specifically, what are (or "were," if you have stopped binge eating) the
processes responsible for your binge eating. To work this out, you will
need to reread Chapter 4. Having done so, ask yourself the following
two questions:

1. *Does dieting contribute to my tendency to binge eat?* If this
seems likely, your dieting will need to be addressed, as described in
the forthcoming Dieting Module (p. 183).
2. *Do concerns about my shape or weight contribute to my binge
eating problem?* If so, these concerns will need to be addressed. How
to do so is described in the Body Image Module (p. 190).

The remainder of the program therefore depends upon your
answers to these two questions because tackling a binge eating problem requires not only addressing the binge eating directly but also
reversing the processes responsible for it. You may need to focus on

> *Tackling a binge eating problem requires not only addressing the binge eating directly but also reversing the processes responsible for it.*

your tendency to diet or your concerns about shape and weight, or you may need to tackle both. If both, then the next question is where to start. Here are two guidelines:

1. If there is just one process to address, say dieting, then go straight to the relevant module.
2. If both dieting and concerns about shape and weight are contributing to your eating problem, start by focusing on the process that seems most important. Then, after 3 or 4 weeks, begin to address the other one as well. In other words, do not embark upon both modules at once. This would be too much to take on.

Meanwhile you will need to continue to practice what you have learned in Steps 1 to 4.

Dieting Module

Step 1: Starting Well
Self-monitoring
Weekly weighing

Step 2: Regular Eating
Establishing a pattern of regular eating
Stopping vomiting and misusing laxatives or diuretics

Step 3: Alternatives to Binge Eating
Substituting alternative activities
Identifying changes in weight

Step 4: Problem Solving
Practicing problem solving

Step 5: Taking Stock
Reviewing progress
Deciding what else needs to be tackled

| **Dieting Module**
Tackling strict dieting | **Body Image Module**
Addressing shape concerns, shape checking, shape avoidance, and feeling fat |

Ending Well
Maintaining progress
Addressing setbacks

To build on your progress and maintain it, you now need to tackle the processes that make you vulnerable to binge. For example, if your binges are triggered primarily by stress, eating at regular intervals, using alternative activities to cope with urges to eat, and efficient problem solving will often be sufficient on their own. On the other hand, if dieting is contributing to your binge eating, then it also needs to be addressed.

In Chapter 4 (p. 41) you learned about three forms of dieting: delaying eating for long periods of time, restricting the overall amount of food eaten, and avoiding eating certain types of food. All three are common among those who binge, and all three tend to encourage binge eating. You may recall that this is particularly true if the dieting is strict, that is, governed by highly specific rules that tend to be applied in an all-or-nothing fashion. Strict dieters tend to impose on themselves a variety of demanding dietary rules, and they respond to any breaking of these rules by giving up and overeating. As a result they alternate between dieting and binge eating, with each encouraging the other.

To determine whether you are a strict dieter, review your monitoring records to get answers to these two groups of questions:

1. *What do I eat between my binges?*
   Am I purposely restricting what I eat? If so, am I attempting to follow any particular dietary regimen (or goals)?
   Am I trying not to eat for long periods of time?
   Am I attempting to limit the overall amount I eat, perhaps by staying below a set calorie limit?
   Am I avoiding particular types of food, ones that I view as fattening or liable to trigger a binge?
   And, most important, am I dieting in an all-or-nothing way, such that if I break my diet I tend to give up and binge?

2. *What are the triggers of my binges?*
   Are they triggered by breaking one of my dietary rules?
   Do they occur if I eat more than I feel I ought to?
   Are they triggered by eating a banned or forbidden food?

If you are dieting, and most especially if you are dieting in a strict way, and if this seems to be triggering your binges, then it is essential that you tackle your dieting. If you don't,

> *It is essential that you continue to practice what you learned in Steps 1 to 4.*

you will remain prone to binge. Below are guidelines for addressing strict dieting. While following these guidelines it is essential that you continue to practice what you learned in Steps 1 through 4.

ADDRESSING STRICT DIETING

The three types of dieting each require their own approach.

Delaying Eating for Long Periods of Time

This was tackled when you established a pattern of regular eating in Step 2. If in the past you were prone not to eat for long periods of time, it is essential that you place great importance on eating at regular intervals, now, and in the longer term. You might want to reread Step 2.

Restricting the Overall Amount You Eat

Imposing strict limits on how much you eat—for example, by setting a calorie limit—must be resisted for two reasons. First, if the limit is extreme, it will inevitably encourage binge eating because it will create a physiological pressure to eat. Certainly any diet that involves eating much less than 1,500 calories a day will have this effect. It will also create a psychological pressure to eat because it will result in preoccupation with food and eating. Second, strict dieters often set themselves very specific dietary goals, and they are prone to binge if they do not meet them. For example, eating anything over 1,500 calories will represent "failure" to someone who is trying to keep to a 1,500 calorie diet.

To tackle this form of dieting, you must first decide whether there is any good reason to restrict your calorie intake. There is no need for most people with binge eating problems to diet; indeed, it is unwise for them to do so since dieting makes them vulnerable to binge. Assuming that there is no good reason for you to diet, you should do your best to stop doing so. You should stop attempting to restrict the overall amount that you eat and, if applicable, stop counting calories. Paradoxically, this may well result in you eating less overall as you will be less prone to binge.

If you are afraid that you will overeat if you stop dieting, you may need guidelines as to what is a "normal" amount to eat. As suggested in Step 2, one option would be to identify people of about your age (and gender) and see what they eat. Alternatively, you could follow the advice on food packages and in recipes. A friend or relative who is helping you with the program could also advise you. Finally, remember that Table 5 (p. 70) specified the approximate calorie needs of adults with various lifestyles.

Trying to Avoid Certain Foods

It is particularly important to tackle this form of dieting ("food avoidance") because it is especially likely to encourage binge eating (see Chapter 4, p. 43).

In principle, food avoidance is the easiest form of dieting to tackle since all you have to do is introduce the avoided foods into your diet. In practice, however, this is easier said than done. For example, you may have become so used to not eating these foods that you are no longer aware that you are avoiding them. The first step therefore is to identify what foods you are avoiding. The best way of doing this may seem odd, but it works. Go to a local supermarket that stocks most types and brands of food, and walk up and down the aisles, writing down in a notebook—other shoppers may think you are an employee!—all the foods that you would be reluctant to eat, either because of the effect they might have on your weight or shape, or because you think eating them might trigger a binge. A typical list is shown in Figure 26. Then, at home, organize this list (often it

Whole milk	Pancakes	Other pastas
Butter	Ice cream	Pizza
Cheese	Milkshakes	Fried chicken
Bread	Candy bars	French fries
Bagels	Soda	Chicken parm
Muffins	Potato chips	Ribs
Cereal	Tortilla chips	Meatloaf
Cookies	Salad dressing	Hotdogs
Cake	Mayonnaise	Hamburgers
Doughnuts	Macaroni salad	Chinese food
Peanut butter	Spaghetti/noodles	

FIGURE 26. A list of foods avoided by someone with bulimia nervosa.

contains 40 or more items) into three or four groups according to the degree of difficulty that you would have starting to eat them.

The next step is to introduce these foods into your diet. Do so by including them in your planned meals and snacks, and do this only on days on which you feel in control over your eating because otherwise they might trigger a binge. Start by introducing foods from the easiest of your groups and focus on them for a couple of weeks. Then move on to the next group, and so on. Within 6 to 8 weeks you should have incorporated most, if not all, of the foods into your diet. (If your list is particularly long, this might seem unlikely. In practice, the introduction of a food often deals with other related foods so that they are addressed at the same time.) It does not matter how much of the food you eat—even a little will do. Generally it is the thought of having eaten the food that triggers a binge rather than concern about the amount eaten.

Some people find doing this easy, but others do not. Either way, it requires sustained practice. You should keep introducing these foods until you no longer find it difficult. The time to stop is when eating these foods no longer unsettles you. Remember, if you are not avoiding any foods, you are much less likely to binge. By introducing your avoided foods you are inoculating yourself against binge eating.

Introducing avoided foods will enhance your control over eating because you will be less prone to binge. Following this advice may require you to eat foods that you regard as fattening or unhealthy. It is important to persist nonetheless. No foods are inherently fattening; it all depends on the amount of them that you eat. Introducing these foods will enhance your control over eating because you will be less prone to binge. As for their unhealthiness, it is preferable to eat these foods in moderation than to binge on them.

Another point worth stressing is that you will not need to eat these foods forever. Rather, as soon as doing so ceases to make you anxious it would be reasonable to cut back somewhat on those generally accepted to be unhealthy—those high in saturated or trans fats (see Chapter 5, p. 69)—although it would be best not to exclude them altogether. You should allow yourself to eat anything at times; nothing should be rigidly banned.

Finally, it is important to recall that some people justify dieting on the grounds that they are vegetarians or have a food allergy. Whatever the justification, any dietary restriction that is at least in part designed to reduce weight or change shape is a form of dieting that needs to be tackled if you are prone to binge.

Addressing Strict Dieting: What to Do

Follow the guidelines for dealing with the three forms of dieting, and assess your progress at each of your review sessions. Remember to consider each form of dieting.

DIETING MODULE REVIEW SESSIONS

At each weekly review session you should study your monitoring records and summary sheet, and ask yourself the two questions below, in addition to those relating to Steps 1 through 4 and, if applicable, the body image module.

1. Am I tackling the three forms of dieting?
   Trying not to eat for long periods of time.
   Trying to restrict the overall amount I eat.
   Trying to avoid certain types of food.

2. Am I tackling eating in front of others? If not, should I be doing so?

If your answer is "No" to either of these questions, you should consider rereading this module. Also, remember to complete your summary sheet each week. *Classify as a "change day" any day on which . . .*

> You monitored accurately.
> You adhered to weekly weighing.
> You did your best to stick to your planned pattern of eating (Step 2).
> You used your list of alternative activities to deal with any urges to eat or vomit (Step 3).
> You practiced problem solving at every available opportunity (Step 4).
> You tackled strict dieting.

WHEN TO MOVE ON

It takes some time to break out of strict dieting, at least a month or two. It is most important to persevere as otherwise you will remain

> *It is most important to persevere as otherwise you will remain vulnerable to binge.*

vulnerable to binge. In the meantime, you may also be addressing your body image, the other module at this stage in the program.

One final point. Do not forget to complete the final module, "Ending Well." It will help to ensure that the changes you have made persist in the long term.

Body Image Module

Step 1: Starting Well
Self-monitoring
Weekly weighing

Step 2: Regular Eating
Establishing a pattern of regular eating
Stopping vomiting and misusing laxatives or diuretics

Step 3: Alternatives to Binge Eating
Substituting alternative activities
Identifying changes in weight

Step 4: Problem Solving
Practicing problem solving

Step 5: Taking Stock
Reviewing progress
Deciding what else needs to be tackled

Dieting Module
Tackling strict dieting

Body Image Module
Addressing shape concerns, shape checking, shape avoidance, and feeling fat

Ending Well
Maintaining progress
Addressing setbacks

Most people who binge are concerned about their shape and weight. Indeed, these concerns may be so strong that their life becomes dominated by them—nothing else is of such importance. As I explained in Chapter 4 (p. 55), this "overconcern" plays a major role in maintaining many people's binge eating problem. When this is the case it must be addressed. The starting point, therefore, is to consider whether you are concerned about your shape or weight, and to what extent.

IDENTIFYING OVERCONCERN
ABOUT SHAPE AND WEIGHT

What does *overconcern* mean? To restate what was said in Chapter 4, it all centers on how you evaluate yourself. Whereas the majority of people evaluate themselves on the basis of how they are performing in various aspects of life (e.g., the quality of their relationships, their performance at work, their athletic accomplishments), people with eating problems judge their self-worth largely, or even exclusively, in terms of their shape and weight and their ability to control them. A good way of illustrating this is to draw a pie chart in which each slice represents an area of life that you value, its size being in proportion to its significance relative to other aspects of your life. Figures 27 and 28 show two such pie charts, one from a young woman with no eating problem and the other from someone with overconcern about shape and weight.

To assess your degree of concern about shape and weight try creating your own pie chart. This involves the following five steps:

1. ***List the things that are important to you in how you evaluate or judge yourself as a person.*** These are the things in which you try to perform well. To give you some ideas, they may include the quality of your relationships and friendships, your performance at work, your level of fitness, and your performance in other areas of life that you value. If you think carefully about this matter, your list may also need to include your shape and weight, assuming they

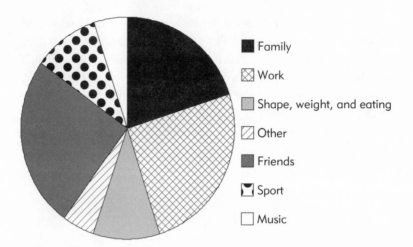

FIGURE 27. The pie chart of a young woman without an eating problem.

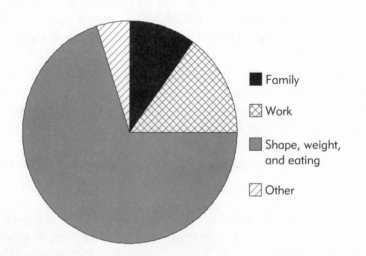

FIGURE 28. The pie chart of a young woman with an eating problem.

are important to how you evaluate yourself as a person. Think hard about your list and be honest with yourself. Do not put things on the list just because you think that they ought to be there.

2. Rank the items on your list in terms of their relative importance. You may find this task difficult but you will discover a hierarchy embedded within your list. It is just a matter of detecting it. A good indication of the importance of a particular feature is how much time and energy you invest in it, as well as how much it would disturb you if this aspect of your life was not going well. For example, how much would it unsettle you if you were told your work was not up to standard? Would this bother you more or less than having an argument with your best friend, being dropped from your sports team, or discovering that an article of clothing was now too tight?

3. Draw your pie chart. Each item on your list should be allocated a slice, and its size should be in proportion to its importance in how you evaluate yourself. Make sure that your pie chart reflects how you really are, rather than how you think you ought to be.

4. Review your pie chart on several occasions over the next week. Is it accurate? Does it represent how you really do evaluate yourself? If it doesn't, make whatever adjustments are appropriate.

5. Examine your pie chart and think about its implications. Is there a slice representing your shape or weight? If so, how big is it? Is it on the large side? If it occupies a third or more of your pie chart, you are almost certainly overconcerned about your shape or weight.

Overconcern about shape and weight is a problem for three main reasons. The first is that it is "risky" being largely dependent on one area of life to feel good about yourself. You have too many eggs in one basket. By this I mean that if this area of life is not going well, you will inevitably feel bad about yourself. The second reason why overconcern about shape and weight is a problem is that there will always be people who seem slimmer or more attractive than you. Therefore, if you judge your self-worth along these lines you will perpetually feel that you are failing. For these two reasons, and the fact that this overconcern plays a major role in maintaining your eating problem, it needs to be addressed. How to do so is the topic of this module.

Even if you are not overconcerned about your shape or weight, you might find aspects of this module of interest and value.

This said, even if you are not overconcerned about shape and weight, you might find aspects of this module of interest and value.

ADDRESSING OVERCONCERN ABOUT SHAPE AND WEIGHT

In principle, there are two ways of reducing overconcern about shape and weight. It is best to do both because they complement each other. The two strategies involve:

1. **Increasing the importance of other areas of your life.**
2. **Decreasing the importance of shape and weight.**

While doing this, it is absolutely essential that you continue to practice what you learned in Steps 1 through 4 of the program.

It is essential that you continue to practice what you learned in Steps 1 to 4.

Increasing the Importance of Other Areas of Your Life

Look again at your pie chart. If you are overconcerned about your shape and weight, this will stand out because there will be a dominant slice representing this overconcern.

Are you being the "real you"? Do you need to get more into your life?

Are there any other obvious problems with your pie chart? It is likely that there are two. First, as a result of having a dominant slice, there is likely to be little room for much else—to put this more clearly, if your pie chart is accurate, it is likely that you do not value much else other than your shape and weight. The second problem is that there may be few other slices (of whatever size) indicating that there is not much else in your life that you value.

Is this right?
Are you happy with this?
Is this the "real you"?

Both of these problems are worth addressing. It is helpful to get more into your life (i.e., more slices) and it is especially helpful if these new areas of life become important to you as a source of self-esteem (i.e., the new slices become big ones).

If you conclude you do need to get more into your life, you should follow the following three steps.

1. Identify potential new activities. Make a list of activities or interests that you used to enjoy, things that you think you might like to try, and things that you have been meaning to do. If you are struggling to come up with ideas, it might help to think what your friends, family, or colleagues do in their spare time. Are any of these activities things that you would like to do? If so, write them down. At this stage it is best not to dismiss anything. Examples might include joining a pottery class, hiking club, or reading group, or going to a film club or dance class.

2. Next, identify one (or possibly two) activities that you would be willing to try in the coming week. It does not matter what the activity is so long as it is not a single, one-time event. Ideally it should take place every week. It is also a good idea to give priority to those activities that involve meeting new people.

3. Commit yourself to engaging in these activities on a regular basis. Do not let obstacles get in your way; problem-solve them if necessary. As a general rule, only abandon an activity once you have tried it on three separate occasions. If then you still do not like it, choose something else from your list.

If you follow these guidelines, your life should gradually become broader and richer—not overnight, of course, but over a matter of months. The "real you" will emerge. And this will become evident in your pie chart. The number of slices will increase and they will occupy more space. But for this to happen the oversized slice, the one representing your shape and weight, will need to shrink. In other words, you will need to decrease the importance that you place on your shape and weight.

Decreasing the Importance of Shape and Weight

The best way of decreasing the importance of shape and weight is to tackle its so-called "expressions." As we discussed in Chapter 4 (p. 58), these are the behaviors and experiences that stem from the overconcern and maintain it (as illustrated in Figure 29). The main ones are body checking, body avoidance, and feeling fat. If they are successfully addressed, this will undermine your overconcern and it will gradually fade.

> *The best way of decreasing the importance of shape and weight is to tackle its three "expressions": shape checking, shape avoidance, and feeling fat.*

To begin this process, you first need to think which of these behaviors and experiences are relevant to you. You might think that this should be obvious, but in practice it often isn't. Many people are unaware of the extent of their shape checking or how often they "feel fat." You will therefore need to do some additional recording—and you may well find this interesting—but before doing this it would be

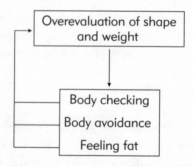

FIGURE 29. The vicious circles maintaining overconcern about shape and weight.

a good idea to read through the rest of this module to get an idea of the types of behavior and feelings you should be looking out for.

Having read through this module, identify two coming days, a workday and a day off from work, and on these two days plan to do some particularly detailed recording. The initial goal will be to identify every time you do or experience the following:

Check your body or aspects of it.
Become particularly aware of your body.
Inspect someone else's body.
Compare your body to that of others.
Avoid your body.
"Feel fat."

To do this, you will need an additional recording sheet for this specific purpose (see Figure 30). Instructions for completing the body image record are given in Table 11. Do your best to do this recording in real time, and do not be surprised or upset if you have a lot to write down. Just try to capture everything, however tempting it might be to leave things off. Figure 31 shows an example of a completed body image record.

Once the 2 days of recording are over you should review your records. If they show that you body check, body compare, body avoid, or "feel fat," and that this is frequent, then it is likely to be fuelling your concerns about your shape and weight, and would therefore be well worth tackling. If several of these phenomena are occurring, as is often the case, begin by tackling one and then after a couple of weeks start addressing another. Tackling the expressions of your overconcern will make you feel much better about yourself and will reliably reduce the extent of your overconcern.

ADDRESSING SHAPE CHECKING

As we discussed in Chapter 4, there are many forms of shape checking. Common ones include studying specific parts of your body in

Time	Checking, etc.	Place	Context, thoughts, and feelings

FIGURE 30. A blank body image record. An enlarged version of this figure may be downloaded from *www.credo-oxford.com*.

TABLE 11. Instructions for completing body image records.

Column 1: Record the time of day.

Column 2: Record every time you check or avoid your body, become particularly aware of your body, compare your body to that of others, inspect someone else's body, or "feel fat." At these times note down exactly what you did and, in brackets, the number of minutes the feeling or behavior lasted.

Column 3: Record where you were at the time.

Column 4: Record the context, thoughts, and feelings that accompanied the behavior or experience.

---

the mirror, pinching or touching your body, assessing the tightness of particular items of clothing or accessories (such as watches or rings), and looking at the extent to which your thighs spread out when you sit down. If you are male you may be more concerned about your build and muscularity (or lack of it) and your checking may therefore focus on this aspect of your body.

Shape checking is unhelpful either when it is extreme (e.g., when it involves scrutiny) or when it is frequent because both forms of checking tend to exaggerate concerns about shape and appearance. Remember the magnifying effect of scrutiny that we discussed in Chapter 4 (see p. 61) and the complexities involved in interpreting what you see in the mirror (see p. 60)? Remember also that if you look for fatness, you will find it.

Scrutiny magnifies, and mirrors are complex.

If you look for fatness, you will find it.

There is also the matter of weight checking, that is, checking the number on the scale. As it happens, you have already addressed this habit and its counterpart, weight avoidance, with the introduction of weekly weighing at the beginning of the program (p. 136). If you were someone who frequently weighed yourself, or avoided knowing your weight, you should now be appreciating the benefits of weekly weighing. Shape checking is approached in much the same way.

Time	Checking, etc.	Place	Context, thoughts, and feelings
6:30	Looked at reflection in mirror (2 mins)	Kitchen	My face looks really fat
7:00	Looked in mirror while getting dressed— kept turning round and round (5 mins) Pinched my fat rolls (2 mins)	Bedroom	Ughh my stomach is so gross
8:30	Checked to see if my backside looks big in this skirt (5 mins)	Bathroom at work	How can I be so fat already? I have only eaten breakfast!
10:00	Looked down at stomach while snacking (2 mins)	Desk	Cannot believe that my stomach is so big—it is making me grossed out to look at it—why can't I just be skinny?
1:15	Watched thin runners in the park (15 mins)	Park	I SHOULD be running like all of these people!
7:30	Read about latest celeb diet (15 mins)	Living room	I am so jealous of these women; if only I had a personal trainer and more willpower!
9:00	Looked at how my thighs spread out when sitting (3 mins)	Living room	I am so sick of this! I hate myself.

FIGURE 31. A completed body image record.

So, having identified your various forms of shape checking, and how often you engage in them, write them down and put them into one or the other of two groups: behaviors that would be best stopped completely, and behaviors that need to be modified. Things that are best stopped completely include anything that is particularly unusual—for example, repeatedly measuring or photographing your body, or studying aspects of yourself. Consider including any form of behavior that would embarrass you if others knew about it. Such behavior is best stopped. Admittedly, it will be difficult doing this, and it will temporarily increase your preoccupation with your shape, but it will get easier quite quickly and ceasing such behavior has many benefits. It will lessen your degree of concern about shape; it will remove a behavior that is secretive and perhaps distressing; and it will improve your self-regard.

Mirror Use

More commonplace forms of shape checking require a different strategy, one's mirror use being the best example. It would not be appropriate or realistic to never look in a mirror as avoidance is as problematic as repeated checking. Instead, the behavior needs to be modified.

As always, the first step is to find out what you are currently doing. Below are the key questions to ask yourself:

How often do I look in the mirror?
How long do I take?
What exactly do I do when looking in the mirror?
What am I trying to find out? (This is an interesting question that merits some thought.)
Can I find it out this way?
At home, how many different mirrors do I use?

These are questions you may have never considered before. Think carefully about them. If you are someone who looks into the mirror a lot, why do you do it? What are you hoping to find out? Unless you have a photographic memory, you won't be able to detect changes in your shape this way. It is better to rely on your weight graph for this purpose.

Now think about the additional questions below, each of which is accompanied by the types of answer I give my patients.

What are good reasons to look in the mirror?
  To check one's hair and clothing.
  Women need a mirror to apply and remove makeup; men need a mirror to shave.

Are there any other good reasons to look in the mirror?
  No. For people with an eating problem there are no reasons to look in the mirror other than those given above.
  Mirrors are "risky" for people with an eating problem. They are best used judiciously.

How many mirrors is it best to have at home?
  One for the face and another full-length one for the body.
  It is best to get rid of the others unless they are purely decorative. It is difficult to avoid excessive mirror use if there are a large number of mirrors around. Full-length mirrors in the bedroom are particularly problematic.

How can I avoid the "magnification" that comes from scrutiny?
  When looking in the mirror, ensure that you do not focus on particular parts of your body, and especially parts that you dislike. Look at the whole of your body including more neutral areas (e.g., hands, feet, knees, hair). In addition, look at the background environment as this helps give you a sense of scale.

What about looking at myself naked in the mirror?
  Not a good idea, unless you are going to admire yourself!
  People with binge eating problems are most unlikely to be admiring themselves. Rather, they tend to focus on disliked parts and scrutinize them.
  It is also not a good idea to dress or undress in front of a mirror.

I need a mirror to help me choose what clothes to wear, especially if I am going out.

Perhaps, but some people spend an inordinate amount of time doing this, trying on three or more outfits. This is typically accompanied by a progressive increase in their dissatisfaction with their appearance and a decline in their self-confidence. If this applies to you, try to choose your outfit before putting it on (e.g., by laying it out on the bed).

Your aim should be to become aware of your mirror use in real time and seriously question yourself before engaging in it. And do the same with regard to other forms of shape checking while keeping in mind the crucial information in Chapter 4 (pp. 60–62). With regard to mirrors, use them judiciously and try to become better at interpreting what you see.

> Use mirrors judiciously and try to become better at interpreting what you see.

ADDRESSING COMPARISON MAKING

Comparison making is a particular form of shape checking that involves repeatedly comparing your body or appearance with that of other people. It includes comparisons with images in newspapers and magazines and with those on the Internet. As we discussed in Chapter 4 (p. 61), what is striking about such comparison making is that it often results in the person concluding that he or she is unattractive relative to others. This conclusion is the result of the inherent bias in the way that the comparison takes place.

If you are prone to repeated comparison making and it makes you feel bad about yourself, this is a habit well worth addressing. To do so, you should follow these steps.

Go over your records and consider how fair your comparison making is and how it makes you feel. Does it lead you to conclude that your body is unattractive relative to others? If so, are there reasons to question this conclusion? Scrutiny may have led you to believe that your body looks "worse" than it actually does, whereas you may be uncritical when evaluating other people—for example, when passing them on the street. Remember that it is difficult to get the same view of someone else's body as you have of your own. Do you ever look down to see how much your stomach bulges out? Have you ever had the same view of anyone else's body? Do you ever study in detail some part of your body? Have you looked at anyone else's in this exact way? Scrutinizing your body is very different from glancing at someone else's. Can you see that there is a bias here? You study your body in detail and from a particular perspective (looking for faults), whereas you look at other peoples' bodies differently and in a way that is less critical.

There is also an additional source of bias. Many people with binge eating problems compare themselves with a select group, those who are unusually attractive or thin.

Start identifying when and how you make comparisons. Record your comparisons on your usual monitoring records along with the context in which they occur. Then go through each instance with the following two questions in mind:

> *Who did I compare myself with, and how did I select him or her?*
> *How did I assess the person, and what aspect did I focus on?*

Explore the possibility that you may choose a biased group to compare yourself with. With this in mind, you can perform an interesting experiment. Walk down a busy street and compare yourself with every third person who passes you (of your gender and approximate age). You are likely to discover that there is much more variation in body shape and attractiveness than you have previously noticed. This is because you have been selectively comparing yourself with unusually slim or attractive people.

Consider whether the way you assess other people differs from the way you assess yourself. Do you subject other people to the same level of scrutiny? Again, an experiment can be revealing when thinking about this. Go to a public changing room at a swimming pool or gym where people are naked or wearing very little. Then select someone (of your gender and approximate age) who you view as reasonably attractive. Next, discretely scrutinize his or her body focusing *exclusively* on the areas that you tend to focus on. Do this for as long as you can . . . but do remember the "discrete" part! You are likely to discover that, on scrutiny, the person's body is not as flawless as you initially thought—that he or she too has a protruding stomach or dimpled flesh.

From now on, question the conclusions that you draw from each episode of comparison making. Ask yourself whether the comparison was truly an accurate and fair one.

If your tendency is to compare yourself with images in the media, try resisting this for the time being. In the intervening period learn about the routine distortion of photographs by newspapers, magazines, and websites. Go on the Internet and explore the topic of "airbrushing." Also, search for "Dove Evolution" and other videos illustrating photoshopping. We all need to learn to take media images with a pinch of salt. Many of them have been manipulated.

ADDRESSING SHAPE AVOIDANCE

As we discussed in Chapter 4 (p. 62), shape avoidance refers to behavior designed to prevent the person from seeing their body and being aware of it. It often includes avoidance of others seeing their body too. It stems from a strong dislike of how their body looks or feels. The major problem with shape avoidance is that it results in assumptions about the body going unchallenged. As a consequence it is self-perpetuating. When extreme it can be profoundly impairing; for example, it leads to some people being unable to socialize normally or to have intimate relationships.

Shape avoidance is best addressed by progressive "exposure." This involves getting used to the sight and feel of your body. This is best done in steps. You should follow the guidelines

It is liberating to free yourself from shape avoidance.

below, moving through the various steps as rapidly as you can. It is liberating to free yourself from shape avoidance. It is far better to know your own body than to avoid it.

> ***If you get dressed and undressed in the dark.*** Begin by putting candles in the bedroom and work your way toward getting dressed with the lights on.
>
> ***If you avoid touching your body.*** Begin by washing yourself in a conscious way. You might want to start by washing yourself with a sponge, focusing on neutral body parts like your feet or hands. You should work toward being able to wash your whole body using your hands.
>
> ***If you try to avoid being aware of your body.*** Do things that increase your body awareness or involve some degree of body exposure. For example, you could apply body lotion on a daily basis; you could have a regular massage; you could go swimming or join a dance class. And try to avoid wearing baggy, formless clothes.

ADDRESSING FEELING FAT

As we discussed in Chapter 4 (p. 63), "feeling fat" is important. Not only is it distressing, but it is common for people to equate feeling fat with being fat, with the result that their concerns about shape and weight are reinforced. And what is especially noteworthy about feeling fat is that the experience fluctuates greatly, both from day to day and within a day. This is quite unlike the overconcern with shape and weight, which tends to be relatively stable (as illustrated in Figure 32).

If you "feel fat" at times and it is a source of distress or it leads you to diet, then the phenomenon needs to be tackled. To do so, you need to learn more about the experience. You need to find out what triggers it, and what else you are feeling at the same time. This is because feeling fat seems to be the result of the mislabeling of unpleasant emotions and bodily experiences. To help you discover what underlies your experiences of feeling fat, follow these four steps.

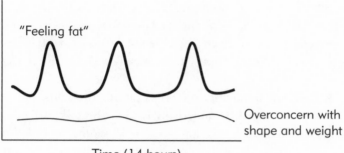

FIGURE 32. "Feeling fat" fluctuates.

1. *Start by identifying the times when you have "peaks" of feeling fat.* Note these down in the last column of your normal monitoring records. Also write down what else you were feeling and doing at these times, and what you were doing in the hour beforehand. Try to capture these times "live" because doing so may uncover important information.

2. *Once you have collected a few examples, which may take several days or a week or so, go through each one during one of your review sessions.* Ask yourself the following two questions with regard to each episode:

> *Was there a trigger? Did something happen in the hour beforehand that might have resulted in me feeling fat?*
> *What else was I feeling or doing at the time that I felt fat?*

Common triggers or accompanying experiences are:
    Feeling bored, sleepy, lonely, depressed, or hungover
    Becoming aware of one's body as a result of shape checking, body comparisons, feeling hot or sweaty, feeling one's body wobble, bodily contact, one's clothes feeling tight
    Feeling full, bloated, or premenstrual

3. *Continue to monitor (in real time) your peaks of feeling fat, but now try to identify their cause there and then.* Each time

you feel fat ask yourself what might have triggered the feeling and what sensations "feeling fat" might be masking. Gradually, a consistent pattern is likely to emerge. Also remind yourself that the feeling has nothing to do with "being fat." Your body will not have suddenly changed.

4. Continue to identify the peaks and their origins, but now practice addressing their underlying cause. This task may involve a simple commonsense solution, such as loosening your clothing, changing into something else, taking a shower, or napping. Or it may involve using the problem-solving approach we practiced in Step 4 (p. 169).

Persist with addressing feeling fat for the next month or so. You will find that the feeling progressively declines in its frequency and intensity. It will also lose its significance as you come to appreciate that it has nothing to do with being fat.

BODY IMAGE REVIEW SESSIONS

At each weekly review session you should study your monitoring records and summary sheet and ask yourself the two questions below in addition to those relating to Steps 1 through 4 and, if applicable, the dieting module.

1. *Am I getting more into my life? Am I doing new things?*
2. *Am I addressing the three main "expressions" of overconcern about shape and weight?*
    Shape checking (including comparison making)
    Shape avoidance
    Feeling fat

Also, remember to complete your summary sheet each week. *Classify as a "change day" any day on which . . .*

You monitored accurately.
You adhered to weekly weighing.

You did your best to stick to your planned pattern of eating (Step 2).

You used your list of alternative activities to deal with any urges to eat or vomit (Step 3).

You practiced problem solving at every available opportunity (Step 4).

You tackled strict dieting (if applicable).

You engaged in a new activity.

You made progress in addressing shape checking, shape avoidance, and feeling fat.

WHEN TO MOVE ON

It is most important to persevere as otherwise you will remain vulnerable to binge.

Changing body image takes months. After all, you are trying to change how you see and evaluate yourself as a person. Do persevere, however, as otherwise you will remain vulnerable to binge. It will be worth it. In the meantime, you may also be addressing your dieting, the other module at this stage in the program.

One final point. Do not forget to complete the final module, "Ending Well." It will help to ensure that the changes you have made persist in the long term.

Ending Well

Step 1: Starting Well
Self-monitoring
Weekly weighing

Step 2: Regular Eating
Establishing a pattern of regular eating
Stopping vomiting and misusing laxatives or diuretics

Step 3: Alternatives to Binge Eating
Substituting alternative activities
Identifying changes in weight

Step 4: Problem Solving
Practicing problem solving

Step 5: Taking Stock
Reviewing progress
Deciding what else needs to be tackled

Dieting Module	Body Image Module
Tackling strict dieting	Addressing shape concerns, shape checking, shape avoidance, and feeling fat

Ending Well
Maintaining progress
Addressing setbacks

Now that you have nearly completed the program, it is time to take stock once again. It is possible that you still have a significant eating problem. If binge eating is continuing to interfere with your quality of life, you should seriously consider getting further help. The options were outlined at the beginning of the program (p. 122). The fact that this program did not help, or did so only to a limited degree, does not mean that the problem cannot be overcome. Far from it. There are many treatment options. Do not give up.

On the other hand, things may have improved and may still be improving. If this is the case, then two final matters need to be considered:

1. How to maintain your progress.
2. How to deal with setbacks.

These two topics are the focus of this final module.

MAINTAINING YOUR PROGRESS

If your binge eating problem has improved slightly or markedly, then you should continue to employ those elements of the program that you found most helpful. In this way you are likely to continue improving. It is especially important to adhere to "regular eating," possibly indefinitely. Keeping up problem solving can be helpful too. Also, you should continue to hold regular review sessions (over the next 3 or so months) to keep an eye on your progress.

There are components of the program you can drop, however. You can stop monitoring if your eating is stable and satisfactory. However, be wary of stopping because you don't want to face up to ongoing difficulties.

Similarly, you can cease weekly weighing if your weight is stable and satisfactory. This said, as part of adopting a healthy lifestyle, it is a good idea to check your weight at regular intervals.

DEALING WITH SETBACKS

The Importance of Realistic Expectations

It is common for people who have stopped binge eating to hope that they will never binge again. While this hope is understandable, it is neither helpful nor realistic. You should regard your eating problem as your Achilles' heel. You will still be prone to react this way at times of difficulty. Just as some people react to stress by becoming depressed or irritable, or by drinking too much, so people who have had an eating problem are liable to start eating differently.

The Triggers of Setbacks

Setbacks are inevitable, and they are especially likely during the weeks and months when you are emerging from an eating problem. They are less likely later on. However, they can occur at any time, even years or decades later. The most likely triggers are as follows:

Adverse events. Stressful events in general, especially those that threaten self-esteem.

Developing a clinical depression. Clinical depressions are particularly prone to trigger a setback.

Shape- or weight-related events. These include a significant increase in weight; an apparent increase in "fatness"; critical comments from others; shape and weight change following pregnancy; and loss of weight due to illness.

Eating-related events. These include restarting dieting, breaking a major remaining dietary rule, and binge eating (i.e., one binge triggering another).

While some of these events and circumstances are outside your control, the most major one is not. It is dieting. To minimize the chances that your binge eating problem will return, do your best not to diet and, most important of all, do not engage in strict dieting (see Chapter 4, p. 44).

Addressing Setbacks

Given that setbacks are inevitable, it is important to have a plan for dealing with them (even if you think this is not necessary in your case). Indeed, how you deal with your setbacks is central to the prevention of relapses.

It is particularly important to distinguish a "lapse" from a "relapse." A *lapse* is a setback or slip, whereas a *relapse* is returning to square one. The two words have different connotations. Implicit in the notion of a lapse is the idea that there can be degrees of deterioration. On the other hand, the notion of a relapse suggests that one is either well or right back to square one. This type of thinking should be familiar by now; it is another example of all-or-nothing (dichotomous) thinking, a thinking style that is common among people who binge.

To minimize the chances of relapsing, it is essential not to mislabel any lapse (or setback) as a relapse because doing so is likely to affect your behavior. If you think you are having a lapse, you are likely to take active steps to get back on track, whereas if you regard yourself as having relapsed, you may well give up and as a result matters will get worse.

There are three aspects to dealing with a lapse:

1. *Spot the problem early.* This is important. The "head in the sand" approach only makes matters worse. If your binge eating has returned or become more frequent, you should act, and act as soon as you can. If you think there is a problem, it is best to assume that this is the case and take steps to do something about it. If you think you might be having a setback, almost certainly you are.

2. *Do the right thing.* Reinstitute the program in this book. Restart monitoring and weekly weighing; force yourself to eat at regular intervals; and engage in whatever other elements of the program that seem relevant. Be your own therapist. Reread the whole of Part II. And do your utmost to resist the temptation to cut back on your eating as this will only make you more prone to binge. And remember to review your progress every few days.

3. Identify and address the trigger of the setback. You need to think what has led to the setback. It may be obvious or it may not. Think long and hard about this. Once you have identified the likely trigger, address it. If relevant, use the problem-solving approach in Step 4 (p. 169).

With this three-pronged approach, you will find that you can nip most lapses in the bud, well before they get a hold. But if you are not succeeding, seriously consider seeking professional help. Guidance for doing so is provided in Appendix I.

APPENDIX I

Obtaining Professional Help
for an Eating Problem

If you think you need outside help for your eating problem or for an associated difficulty, then it is important to see someone who is competent to provide it. Finding such a professional is not necessarily straightforward. It may be that your physician or another health care professional can recommend someone suitable. If not, you might want to go on the Internet to explore the various options. A good starting point is the Academy for Eating Disorders (*www.aedweb. org*), a professional organization devoted to eating disorder research, education, treatment, and prevention. It provides guidance for identifying suitable professionals. It also provides links to other similar organizations in the United States and abroad.

APPENDIX II

Calculating Your Body Mass Index

The body mass index (BMI) is a useful way of determining whether someone is underweight, normal weight, or overweight. It is simply a number representing a person's weight adjusted for his or her height. Specifically it is weight in kilograms divided by height in meters squared—that is, weight/(height × height). In general, the BMI applies to adults of both sexes between the ages of 18 and 60, an exception being those with a particularly large muscle mass (e.g., many athletes).

The chart on the following pages (see Figure 33) can be used to identify your BMI. Look along the top to find your height and then look down the left-hand column to find your weight. Where your height and weight intersect in the table is your BMI.

Alternatively, you can use one of the many BMI calculators on the Internet (e.g., *www.cdc.gov/healthyweight/assessing/bmi*).

The following BMI thresholds are used to classify people as underweight, healthy weight, overweight, or having obesity.

Underweight   Below 18.5
Healthy weight   18.5 to 24.9
Overweight   25.0 to 29.9
Obese   30.0 and above

Note that these thresholds are based on health risks, not appearance.

If your BMI is 25.0 or above, you are at increased risk of a wide range of health problems, the main ones being the following:

Diabetes
Heart disease and high blood pressure
Stroke
Certain cancers
Osteoarthritis
Pregnancy complications

In Appendix III I discuss what to do if your BMI is 25.0 or above (i.e., if you are overweight) and you have a binge eating problem.

HEIGHT (inches, meters)

Lbs	Kg	Inches / Meters / Stones	58.0 / 1.47	59.0 / 1.50	60.0 / 1.52	61.0 / 1.55	62.0 / 1.57	63.0 / 1.60	64.0 / 1.63	65.0 / 1.65	66.0 / 1.68	67.0 / 1.70	68.0 / 1.73	69.0 / 1.75	70.0 / 1.78	71.0 / 1.80	72.0 / 1.83	73.0 / 1.85	74.0 / 1.88	75.0 / 1.91	76.0 / 1.93
80.0	36.3	5st 10lb	16.8	16.1	15.7	15.1	14.7	14.2	13.7	13.3	12.9	12.6	12.1	11.9	11.5	11.2	10.8	10.6	10.3	10.0	9.7
85.0	38.6	6st 1lb	17.9	17.2	16.7	16.1	15.7	15.1	14.5	14.2	13.7	13.4	12.9	12.6	12.2	11.9	11.5	11.3	10.9	10.6	10.4
90.0	40.9	6st 6lb	18.9	18.2	17.7	17.0	16.6	16.0	15.4	15.0	14.5	14.2	13.7	13.4	12.9	12.6	12.2	12.0	11.6	11.2	11.0
95.0	43.1	6st 11lb	19.9	19.2	18.7	17.9	17.5	16.8	16.2	15.8	15.3	14.9	14.4	14.1	13.6	13.3	12.9	12.6	12.2	11.8	11.6
100.0	45.5	7st 2lb	21.1	20.2	19.7	18.9	18.5	17.8	17.1	16.7	16.1	15.7	15.2	14.9	14.4	14.0	13.6	13.3	12.9	12.5	12.2
105.0	47.7	7st 7lb	22.1	21.2	20.6	19.9	19.4	18.6	18.0	17.5	16.9	16.5	15.9	15.6	15.1	14.7	14.2	13.9	13.5	13.1	12.8
110.0	50.0	7st 12lb	23.1	22.2	21.6	20.8	20.3	19.5	18.8	18.4	17.7	17.3	16.7	16.3	15.8	15.4	14.9	14.6	14.1	13.7	13.4
115.0	52.3	8st 3lb	24.2	23.2	22.6	21.8	21.2	20.4	19.7	19.2	18.5	18.1	17.5	17.1	16.5	16.1	15.6	15.3	14.8	14.3	14.0
120.0	54.5	8st 8lb	25.2	24.2	23.6	22.7	22.1	21.3	20.5	20.0	19.3	18.9	18.2	17.8	17.2	16.8	16.3	15.9	15.4	14.9	14.6
125.0	56.8	8st 13lb	26.3	25.2	24.6	23.6	23.0	22.2	21.4	20.9	20.1	19.7	19.0	18.5	17.9	17.5	17.0	16.6	16.1	15.6	15.2
130.0	59.1	9st 4lb	27.3	26.3	25.6	24.6	24.0	23.1	22.2	21.7	20.9	20.4	19.7	19.3	18.7	18.2	17.6	17.3	16.7	16.2	15.9
135.0	61.4	9st 9lb	28.4	27.3	26.6	25.6	24.9	24.0	23.1	22.6	21.8	21.2	20.5	20.0	19.4	19.0	18.3	17.9	17.4	16.8	16.5
140.0	63.6	10st	29.4	28.3	27.5	26.5	25.8	24.8	23.9	23.4	22.5	22.0	21.3	20.8	20.1	19.6	19.0	18.6	18.0	17.4	17.1
145.0	65.9	10st 5lb	30.5	29.3	28.5	27.4	26.7	25.7	24.8	24.2	23.3	22.8	22.0	21.5	20.8	20.3	19.7	19.3	18.6	18.1	17.7
150.0	68.2	10st 10lb	31.6	30.3	29.5	28.4	27.7	26.6	25.7	25.1	24.2	23.6	22.8	22.3	21.5	21.0	20.4	19.9	19.3	18.7	18.3
155.0	70.5	11st 1lb	32.6	31.3	30.5	29.3	28.6	27.5	26.5	25.9	25.0	24.4	23.6	23.0	22.3	21.8	21.1	20.6	19.9	19.3	18.9
160.0	72.7	11st 6lb	33.6	32.3	31.5	30.3	29.5	28.4	27.4	26.7	25.8	25.2	24.3	23.7	22.9	22.4	21.7	21.2	20.6	19.9	19.5
165.0	75.0	11st 11lb	34.7	33.3	32.5	31.2	30.4	29.3	28.2	27.5	26.6	26.0	25.1	24.5	23.7	23.1	22.4	21.9	21.2	20.6	20.1
170.0	77.3	12st 2lb	35.8	34.4	33.5	32.2	31.4	30.2	29.1	28.4	27.4	26.7	25.8	25.2	24.4	23.9	23.1	22.6	21.9	21.2	20.8
175.0	79.5	12st 7lb	36.8	35.3	34.4	33.1	32.3	31.1	29.9	29.2	28.2	27.5	26.6	26.0	25.1	24.5	23.7	23.2	22.5	21.8	21.3
180.0	81.8	12st 12lb	37.9	36.4	35.4	34.0	33.2	32.0	30.8	30.0	29.0	28.3	27.3	26.7	25.8	25.2	24.4	23.9	23.1	22.4	22.0

WEIGHT (pounds, kg, or stones and pounds)

Weight (lb)	Stones/lb	kg																			
185.0	13st 3lb	84.1	38.9	37.4	36.4	35.0	34.1	32.9	31.7	30.9	29.8	29.1	28.1	27.5	26.5	26.0	25.1	24.6	23.8	23.1	22.6
190.0	13st 8lb	86.4	40.0	38.4	37.4	36.0	35.1	33.8	32.5	31.7	30.6	29.9	28.9	28.2	27.3	26.7	25.8	25.2	24.4	23.7	23.2
195.0	13st 13lb	88.6	41.0	39.4	38.3	36.9	35.9	34.6	33.3	32.5	31.4	30.7	29.6	28.9	28.0	27.3	26.5	25.9	25.1	24.3	23.8
200.0	14st 4lb	90.9	42.1	40.4	39.3	37.8	36.9	35.5	34.2	33.4	32.2	31.5	30.4	29.7	28.7	28.1	27.1	26.6	25.7	24.9	24.4
205.0	14st 9lb	93.2	43.1	41.4	40.3	38.8	37.8	36.4	35.1	34.2	33.0	32.2	31.1	30.4	29.4	28.8	27.8	27.2	26.4	25.5	25.0
210.0	15st	95.5	44.2	42.4	41.3	39.8	38.7	37.3	35.9	35.1	33.8	33.0	31.9	31.2	30.1	29.5	28.5	27.9	27.0	26.2	25.6
215.0	15st 5lb	97.7	45.2	43.4	42.3	40.7	39.6	38.2	36.8	35.9	34.6	33.8	32.6	31.9	30.8	30.2	29.2	28.5	27.6	26.8	26.2
220.0	15st 10lb	100.0	46.3	44.4	43.3	41.6	40.6	39.1	37.6	36.7	35.4	34.6	33.4	32.7	31.6	30.9	29.9	29.2	28.3	27.4	26.8
225.0	16st 1lb	102.3	47.3	45.5	44.3	42.6	41.5	40.0	38.5	37.6	36.2	35.4	34.2	33.4	32.3	31.6	30.5	29.9	28.9	28.0	27.5
230.0	16st 6lb	104.5	48.4	46.4	45.2	43.5	42.4	40.8	39.3	38.4	37.0	36.2	34.9	34.1	33.0	32.3	31.2	30.5	29.6	28.6	28.1
235.0	16st 11lb	106.8	49.4	47.5	46.2	44.5	43.3	41.7	40.2	39.2	37.8	37.0	35.7	34.9	33.7	33.0	31.9	31.2	30.2	29.3	28.7
240.0	17st 2lb	109.1	50.5	48.5	47.2	45.4	44.3	42.6	41.1	40.1	38.7	37.8	36.5	35.6	34.4	33.7	32.6	31.9	30.9	29.9	29.3
245.0	17st 7lb	111.4	51.6	49.5	48.2	46.4	45.2	43.5	41.9	40.9	39.5	38.5	37.2	36.4	35.2	34.4	33.3	32.5	31.5	30.5	29.9
250.0	17st 12lb	113.6	52.6	50.5	49.2	47.3	46.1	44.4	42.8	41.7	40.2	39.3	38.0	37.2	35.9	35.1	33.9	33.2	32.1	31.1	30.5
255.0	18st 3lb	115.9	53.6	51.5	50.2	48.2	47.0	45.3	43.6	42.6	41.1	40.2	38.7	38.0	36.6	35.8	34.6	33.9	32.8	31.8	31.1
260.0	18st 8lb	118.2	54.7	52.5	51.2	49.2	48.0	46.2	44.5	43.4	41.9	40.9	39.5	38.6	37.3	36.5	35.3	34.5	33.4	32.4	31.7
265.0	18st 13lb	120.5	55.8	53.6	52.2	50.2	48.9	47.1	45.4	44.3	42.7	41.7	40.3	39.3	38.0	37.2	36.0	35.2	34.1	33.0	32.3
270.0	19st 4lb	122.7	56.8	54.5	53.1	51.1	49.8	47.9	46.2	45.1	43.5	42.5	41.0	40.1	38.7	37.9	36.6	35.9	34.7	33.6	32.9
275.0	19st 9lb	125.0	57.8	55.6	54.1	52.0	50.7	48.8	47.0	45.9	44.3	43.3	41.8	40.8	39.5	38.6	37.3	36.5	35.4	34.3	33.6
280.0	20st	127.3	58.9	56.6	55.1	53.0	51.6	49.7	47.9	46.8	45.1	44.0	42.5	41.6	40.2	39.3	38.0	37.2	36.0	34.9	34.2
285.0	20st 5lb	129.5	59.9	57.6	56.1	53.9	52.5	50.6	48.7	47.6	45.9	44.8	43.3	42.3	40.9	40.0	38.7	37.8	36.6	35.5	34.8
290.0	20st 10lb	131.8	61.0	58.6	57.0	54.9	53.5	51.5	49.6	48.4	46.7	45.6	44.0	43.0	41.6	40.7	39.4	38.5	37.3	36.1	35.4
295.0	21st 1lb	134.1	62.1	59.6	58.0	55.8	54.4	52.4	50.5	49.3	47.5	46.4	44.8	43.8	42.3	41.4	40.0	39.2	37.9	36.8	36.0
300.0	21st 6lb	136.4	63.1	60.6	59.0	56.8	55.3	53.3	51.3	50.1	48.3	47.2	45.6	44.5	43.1	42.1	40.7	39.9	38.6	37.4	36.6

WEIGHT (pounds, kg, or stones and pounds)

FIGURE 33. BMI chart.

219

APPENDIX III

If You Are Also Overweight

Some people with binge eating problems are also overweight (a BMI of 25.0 or more; see Appendix II). The relationship between binge eating and obesity is complex: The two problems interact and exacerbate each other (see Chapter 6). Binge eating contributes to the maintenance of obesity, and it complicates its treatment. Conversely, those treatments for obesity that involve strict dieting tend to make binge eating problems worse. In general, if you have both a binge eating problem and a weight problem, it is best to address the eating problem first.

If you have both a binge eating problem and a weight problem, it is best to address the eating problem first.

When it comes to addressing a weight problem, an important first step is to see a physician or other health care professional in order to discuss your health, your BMI, and your desire to lose weight. He or she will be able to comment on the advisability of losing weight and an appropriate weight loss goal.

The next step is to identify a weight loss program. Unfortunately, not all programs can be recommended. Some make unrealistic claims and some endorse unhealthy practices. It is therefore important to check out any program before committing yourself to it. It is possible that your physician or health care professional may be able to recommend one.

If you are unsure how to proceed, it is worth looking at the National Institutes of Health websites. They have a "Weight-Control

Information Network" (*http://win.niddk.nih.gov*) that provides up-to-date information on weight control together with a large number of useful publications including an excellent one called *Choosing a Safe and Successful Weight-Loss Program.*

An important point to keep in mind when selecting a weight loss program is whether it is likely to worsen, or bring back, your binge eating problem. Discuss this matter with the people who run the program. You should certainly avoid weight loss programs that encourage strict dieting or forbid the consumption of particular foods.

You should avoid weight loss programs that encourage strict dieting or forbid the consumption of particular foods.

APPENDIX IV

Tackling "Other Problems"

It is not uncommon for people with eating problems to have other difficulties. These vary in nature but often involve problems with mood, self-esteem, and assertiveness; problems with perfectionism; and unsatisfactory relationships and life circumstances. What should be done about these accompanying difficulties? The answer depends upon their seriousness and your circumstances. If the problem is a major concern, you should seek professional advice, if only to have it assessed. This particularly applies if your mood is unusually low and has been like this for some weeks. It is not uncommon for clinical depressions to coexist with binge eating problems. If the problem does not merit seeking professional advice, you could try to tackle it yourself using one of the following self-help programs.

RECOMMENDED SELF-HELP BOOKS

There are books, similar to this one, that provide clear, sensible guidelines for overcoming many of the difficulties that commonly accompany binge eating problems. These are listed below classified by the topics that they address. It is a select list based on my knowledge of the available books and that of trusted experts. No doubt there are many other excellent books that I could have listed, but had I done so I would have strayed away from the books that I know or have had recommended. All the books are readily available and in each case the latest edition is cited.

General

Butler, G., & Hope, T. (2007). *Managing your mind* (2nd ed.). New York: Oxford University Press.

Unlike the books below, this one covers a broad range of topics including problems with mood, relationships, substance use, sleep, studying, making decisions, and much more. Its strength is its breadth. It is a good first stop if you think you might have a problem and would like to learn more about it and its possible solutions.

Lack of Assertiveness

Alberti, R., & Emmons, M. (2008). *Your perfect right.* Atascadero, CA: Impact.

This is a bestseller and deservedly so. It addresses both over- and underassertiveness in an engaging and extremely practical way. Few people would not benefit from reading this book.

Perfectionism

Antony, M. M., & Swinson, R. P. (2008). *When perfect isn't good enough.* Oakland, CA: New Harbinger.

Another long-established book that has survived the test of time. Written by two experts in the field, this book addresses the often overlooked problem of having excessively high standards. If you suspect that you might have this tendency (and others would agree), then this book is for you.

Low Self-Esteem

Fennell, M. (2009). *Overcoming low self-esteem.* London: Robinson.

Written by an expert on self-esteem, this book helps readers explore their self-esteem and what it is founded on. It then goes on to recommend ways of bolstering one's self-regard using strategies and techniques from cognitive behavior therapy.

Marital Conflict

Gottman, J., & Silver, N. (2007). *The seven principles for making marriage work.* London: Orion.

This book has been recommended by colleagues whose opinion I trust. It provides straightforward, evidence-based guidelines for improving marital relationships, the focus being primarily on restoring the core relationship.

APPENDIX V

A Note for Relatives and Friends

Overcoming Binge Eating provides an account of what is known about binge eating problems and their treatment (Part I) together with a detailed step-by-step self-help program based on the most effective treatment available (Part II).

If you have bought this book because you are concerned that a relative or friend might have a binge eating problem, then the main descriptive chapters (Chapters 1 and 4) should clarify matters. And if you are concerned about the physical effects of binge eating problems, read Chapter 5. Treatment is discussed in Chapter 8.

Perhaps you think your relative or friend has a binge eating problem, but the matter has never been discussed. This is a difficult situation since it is obviously their right to decide whether they want to talk about it or not. Nevertheless, it does seem reasonable to ensure that they are well informed. An appropriate initial step is therefore to encourage the person to read this book. How this can best be achieved will depend on the exact circumstances and may require considerable sensitivity on your part. Keep in mind that binge eating problems are associated with shame and self-recrimination so being "found out" can come as a considerable shock.

If the problem is in the open, the issue may be how you can help. This will depend on whether your relative or friend wants to change. If ambivalence is a problem, you might want to suggest that he or she read the section "Why Change?" at the beginning of Part II (p.

119). However, if he or she already has a desire to change, you might together review the various treatment options (see p. 122) to decide which would be best. If the decision is to seek professional treatment, then you can help by facilitating this goal. And once a competent therapist has been identified (for guidance, see Appendix I), it may well be appropriate to find out what role, if any, you should take. It is important to stress, however, that you should avoid becoming over-involved. Sometimes the most caring thing that you can do is to be there in the background and make yourself available when needed.

If the decision is to use the self-help program in Part II, then a backseat role is certainly best. It is a good idea to read Part I and familiarize yourself with Part II so that you know what the program involves, but it will be up to your relative or friend to decide how you can be of most assistance to him or her. Remember, the program involves the person concerned becoming his or her own therapist. You may have no other role than being available to provide support or advice at difficult times. This can be a difficult part to play. You may feel tempted to step in when you should not, or you could be asked to help at an inconvenient time.

Your relative or friend may feel discouraged or even hopeless at times. They may feel that they will never overcome their binge eating problem. If they share such feelings with you, help them review their progress in a balanced way, and make sure that all their achievements are highlighted as they can get overlooked. Point out all signs of progress and provide as much encouragement as you can.

One other point is worth making. You may feel that the program is too simple to work. This is not the case. It has been extensively tested—possibly better tested than any other self-help program (for any problem)—and it has been shown to be effective (see Chapter 8). Try not to undermine the program. Instead, suspend any misgivings and support your relative or friend as best you can.

APPENDIX VI

A Note for Therapists

As a therapist helping someone with a binge eating problem, you can take one of two roles with respect to this self-help program. You can directly help the person follow the program ("guided self-help"; see p. 113), or you can provide a completely different form of therapy while at the same time supporting his or her use of the program. In the latter case you may decide to have little or no direct involvement with its use. But even with this approach I suggest that you familiarize yourself with the program in case it clashes in any way with the help that you are providing.

An extensive and robust body of research in the United States and elsewhere has shown that guided self-help is a potent way of helping those with binge eating problems. It is certainly an excellent first step. It involves the person following the program supported by regular sessions with you. These can be quite brief (less than 30 minutes long) and need not be scheduled every week, although it is best to start this way. Since the program involves the person becoming his or her own therapist, your role differs from that in more conventional forms of therapy. In guided self-help you serve as a "facilitator." Your primary role is to monitor the person's progress, provide encouragement and, at times of difficulty, help him or her to identify solutions from within the program. To do this, you need to be thoroughly familiar with it.

An important aspect of your role in guided self-help is to keep the person motivated. Reviewing the monitoring records at the beginning of each session is a good way of achieving this goal since it provides a means of identifying and highlighting progress. Another aspect of your role is to ensure that the person moves through the program at an appropriate pace. Some want to go too fast; others want to go too slow. The sections titled "When to Move On" provide clear guidelines for when it is appropriate to progress from one step to the next. A third role is to keep the person focused on the goal of the program, which is to overcome his or her binge eating problem. While fulfilling these roles you must stay in the background, an unfamiliar stance for some therapists. Remember, guided self-help is a form of "self-help." The person with the binge eating problem must remain in charge and be his or her own therapist.

There is one other way that this book can be used. Since it provides sound information and advice, it can supplement more conventional approaches to treatment. For example, it is widely employed as an adjunct to pharmacotherapy, cognitive behavior therapy, and other psychological treatments. In addition, it is often used by inpatient programs.

Further Reading

Any list of further reading will rapidly become out of date. For this reason the list below is restricted to key sources that are likely to stand the test of (some) time. Readers wanting to obtain more up-to-date information should use the Internet for this purpose. The obvious search terms will work well.

There are two main scientific journals devoted to the topic of eating disorders:

International Journal of Eating Disorders
European Eating Disorders Review

The websites of these journals are worth examining. There is also a new one, *Journal of Eating Disorders*. In addition, articles on eating disorders are regularly published in the leading medical, psychiatric, and psychological journals, all of which are indexed on the Internet.

There are many books on eating disorders. Below are some key reference books for professionals.

Agras, W. S. (Ed.). (2010). *The Oxford handbook of eating disorders*. New York: Oxford University Press.

Fairburn, C. G. (2008). *Cognitive behavior therapy and eating disorders*. New York: Guilford Press.

Grilo, C. M. (2006). *Eating and weight disorders*. New York: Psychology Press.

Grilo, C. M., & Mitchell, J. E. (Eds.). (2010). *The treatment of eating disorders*. New York: Guilford Press.

Le Grange, D., & Lock, J. (Eds.). (2011). *Eating disorders in children and adolescents*. New York: Guilford Press.

There follows sources of further information of relevance to each section of this book. The majority of the citations refer to review articles. They are not exhaustive.

THIS BOOK AND HOW TO USE IT

Fairburn, C. G., Cooper, Z., & Shafran, R. (2003). Cognitive behaviour therapy for eating disorders: A "transdiagnostic" theory and treatment. *Behaviour Research and Therapy, 41,* 509–528.

Fairburn, C. G., Cooper, Z., Doll, H. A., O'Connor, M. E., Bohn, K., Hawker, D. M., et al. (2009). Transdiagnostic cognitive behavioral therapy for patients with eating disorders: A two-site trial with 60-week follow-up. *American Journal of Psychiatry, 166,* 311–319.

Wilson, G. T., & Zandberg, L. J. (2012). Cognitive-behavioral guided self-help for eating disorders: Effectiveness and scalability. *Clinical Psychology Review, 32,* 343–357.

Randomized Controlled Studies of Overcoming Binge Eating

Carter, J. C., & Fairburn, C. G. (1998). Cognitive-behavioral self-help for binge eating disorder: A controlled effectiveness study. *Journal of Consulting and Clinical Psychology, 66,* 616–623.

DeBar, L., Striegel-Moore, R., Wilson, G. T., Perrin, N., Yarborough, B. J., Dickerson, J., et al. (2011). Guided self-help treatment for recurrent binge eating: Replication and extension. *Psychiatric Services, 62,* 367–373.

Dunn, E. C., Neighbors, C., & Larimer, M. E. (2006). Motivational enhancement therapy and self-help treatment for binge eaters. *Psychology of Addictive Behaviors, 20,* 44–52.

Ghaderi, A. (2006). Attrition and outcome in self-help treatment for bulimia nervosa and binge eating disorder: A constructive replication. *Eating Behaviors, 7,* 300–308.

Ghaderi, A., & Scott, B. (2003). Pure and guided self-help for full and sub-threshold bulimia nervosa and binge eating disorder. *British Journal of Clinical Psychology, 42,* 257–269.

Grilo, C. M., & Masheb, R. M. (2005). A randomized controlled comparison of guided self-help, cognitive behavioral therapy and behavioral weight loss for binge eating disorder. *Behaviour Research and Therapy, 43,* 1509–1525.

Grilo, C. M., Masheb, R. M., & Salant, S. L. (2005). Cognitive behavioral therapy guided self-help and orlistat for the treatment of binge eating disorder: A randomized, double-blind, placebo-controlled trial. *Biological Psychiatry, 57,* 1193–1201.

Ljotsson, B., Lundin, C., Mitsell, K., Carlbring, P., Ramklint, M., & Ghaderi, A. (2007). Remote treatment of bulimia nervosa and binge eating disorder: A randomized trial of Internet-assisted cognitive behavioral therapy. *Behaviour Research and Therapy, 45,* 649–661.

Loeb, K. L., Wilson, G. T., Gilbert, J. S., & Labouvie, E. (2000). Guided and unguided self-help for binge eating. *Behaviour Research and Therapy, 30,* 259–272.

Mitchell, J. E., Agras, S., Crow, S., Halmi, K., Fairburn, C. G., Bryson, S., et al. (2011). Stepped care and cognitive behavioral therapy for bulimia nervosa: Randomised trial. *British Journal of Psychiatry, 198,* 391–397.

Palmer, R. L., Birchall, H., McGrain, L., & Sullivan, V. (2002). Self-help for bulimic disorders: A randomized controlled trial comparing minimal guidance with face-to-face or telephone guidance. *British Journal of Psychiatry, 181,* 230–235.

Ramklint, M., Jeansson, M., Holmgren, S., & Ghaderi, A. (2012). Guided self-help as the first step for bulimic symptoms: Implementation of a stepped-care model with specialized psychiatry. *International Journal of Eating Disorders, 45,* 70–78.

Striegel-Moore, R. H., Wilson, G. T., DeBar, L., Perrin, N., Lynch, F., Rosselli, F., et al. (2010). Cognitive behavioral guided self-help for the treatment of recurrent binge eating. *Journal of Consulting and Clinical Psychology, 78,* 312–321.

Walsh, B. T., Fairburn, C. G., Mickley, D., Sysko, R., & Parides, M. K. (2004). Treatment of bulimia nervosa in a primary care setting. *American Journal of Psychiatry, 161,* 556–561.

Wilson, G. T., Wilfley, D. E., Agras, W. S., & Bryson, S. W. (2010). Psychological treatments for binge eating disorder. *Archives of General Psychiatry, 67,* 94–101.

PART I

Chapter 1

Fairburn, C. G. (2008). The transdiagnostic view and the cognitive behavioral theory. In C. G. Fairburn, *Cognitive behavior therapy and eating disorders.* New York: Guilford Press.

Walsh, B. T. (2011). The importance of eating behavior in eating disorders. *Physiology and Behavior, 104,* 525–529.

Chapter 2

American Psychiatric Association. (2013). *Diagnostic and statistical manual of mental disorders* (fifth edition). Arlington, VA: American Psychiatric Association.

Gordon, K. H., Holm-Denoma, J. M., Crosby, R. D., & Wonderlich, S. A. (2010). The classification of eating disorders. In W. S. Agras (Ed.), *The Oxford handbook of eating disorders.* New York: Oxford University Press.

Vander Wal, J. S. (2012). Night eating syndrome: A critical review of the literature. *Clinical Psychology Review, 32,* 49–59.

Wonderlich, S. A., Gordon, K. H., Mitchell, J. E., Crosby, R. D., & Engel, S. G. (2009). The validity and clinical utility of binge eating disorder. *International Journal of Eating Disorders, 42,* 687–705.

Chapter 3

Keel, P. K. (2010). Epidemiology and course of eating disorders. In W. S. Agras (Ed.), *The Oxford handbook of eating disorders.* New York: Oxford University Press.

Levine, M. P., & Smolak, L. (2010). Cultural influences on body image and the eating disorders. In W. S. Agras (Ed.), *The Oxford handbook of eating disorders.* New York: Oxford University Press.

Norris, M. L., Bondy, S. J., & Pinhas, L. (2011). Epidemiology of eating disorders in children and adolescents. In D. Le Grange & J. Lock (Eds.), *Eating disorders in children and adolescents.* New York: Guilford Press.

Woodside, D. B., Garfinkel, P. E., Lin, E., Goering, P., Kaplan, A. S., Goldbloom, D. S., et al. (2001). Comparisons of men with full or partial eating disorders, men without eating disorders, and women with eating disorders in the community. *American Journal of Psychiatry, 158,* 570–574.

Chapter 4

Fairburn, C. G. (2008). The transdiagnostic view and the cognitive behavioral theory. In C. G. Fairburn, *Cognitive behavior therapy and eating disorders.* New York: Guilford Press.

Hart, S., Abraham, S., Franklin, R. C., & Russell, J. (2011). The reasons why eating disorder patients drink. *European Eating Disorder Review, 19,* 121–128.

Jenkins, P. E., Hoste, R. R., Meyer, C., & Blissett, J. M. (2011). Eating disorders and quality of life: A review of the literature. *Clinical Psychology Review, 31*, 113–121.

Masheb, R. M., Grilo, C. M., & White, M. A. (2011). An examination of eating patterns in community women with bulimia nervosa and binge eating disorder. *International Journal of Eating Disorders, 44*, 616–624.

Chapter 5

Bessesen, D. H. (2011). Regulation of body weight: What is the regulated parameter? *Physiology and Behavior, 104*, 599–607.

Mehler, P. S., Birmingham, C. L., Crow, S. J., & Jahraus, J. P. (2010). Medical complications of eating disorders. In C. M. Grilo & J. E. Mitchell (Eds.), *The treatment of eating disorders*. New York: Guilford Press.

Painter, R. C., Roseboom, T. J., & Bleker, O. P. (2005). Prenatal exposure to the Dutch Famine and disease in later life: An overview. *Reproductive Toxicology, 20*, 345–352.

Pond, C. M. (1998). *The fats of life*. Cambridge, U.K.: Cambridge University Press.

Ravelli, A. C., van der Meulen, J. H. P., Osmond, C., Barker, D. J. P., & Bleker, O. P. (1999). Obesity at the age of 50 in men and women exposed to famine prenatally. *American Journal of Clinical Nutrition, 70*, 811–816.

Roberto, C.A., Mayer, L. E., Brickman, A. M., Baines, A., Muraskin, J., Yeung, L. K., et al. (2011). Brain tissue volume changes following weight gain in adults with anorexia nervosa. *International Journal of Eating Disorders, 44*, 406–411.

Roseboom, T. J., van der Meulen, J. H. P., Osmond, C., Barker, D. J., Ravelli, A. C., Schroeder-Tanka, J. M., et al. (2000). Coronary heart disease after prenatal exposure to the Dutch famine, 1944–45. *Heart, 84*, 595–598.

Chapter 6

Bettle, N., Bettle, O., Neumärker, U., & Neumärker, K.-J. (1998). Adolescent ballet school students: Their quest for body weight change. *Psychopathology, 31*, 153–159.

Clarke, T. K., Weiss, A. R. D., & Berrettini, W. H. (2012). The genetics of anorexia nervosa. *Clinical Pharmacology and Therapeutics, 91,* 181–188.

Jacobi, C., & Fittig, E. (2010). Psychosocial risk factors for eating disorders. In W. S. Agras (Ed.), *The Oxford handbook of eating disorders.* New York: Oxford University Press.

Levine, M. P., & Smolak, L. (2010). Cultural influences on body image and the eating disorders. In W. S. Agras (Ed.), *The Oxford handbook of eating disorders.* New York: Oxford University Press.

Racine, S. E., Root, T. L., Klump, K. L., & Bulik, C. M. (2011). Environmental and genetic risk factors for eating disorders: A developmental perspective. In D. Le Grange & J. Lock (Eds.), *Eating disorders in children and adolescents.* New York: Guilford Press.

Ringham, R., Klump, K., Kaye, W., Stone, D., Libman, S., Stowe, S., et al. (2006). Eating disorder symptomatology among ballet dancers. *International Journal of Eating Disorders, 39,* 503–508.

Wade, T. D. (2010). Genetic influences on eating and eating disorders. In W. S. Agras (Ed.), *The Oxford handbook of eating disorders.* New York: Oxford University Press.

Chapter 7

Wilson, G. T. (2010). Eating disorders, obesity and addiction. *European Eating Disorders Review, 18,* 341–351.

Ziauddeen, H., Farooqi, S., & Fletcher, P. C. (2012). Obesity and the brain: How convincing is the addiction model? *Nature Reviews: Neuroscience, 13,* 279–286.

Chapter 8

Fairburn, C. G. (2008). *Cognitive behavior therapy and eating disorders.* New York: Guilford Press.

Hay, P. J., & Claudino, A. de M. (2010). Evidence-based treatment for the eating disorders. In W. S. Agras (Ed.), *The Oxford handbook of eating disorders.* New York: Oxford University Press.

Ramklint, M., Jeansson, M., Holmgren, S., & Ghaderi, A. (2012). Guided self-help as the first step for bulimic symptoms: Implementation of a stepped-care model with specialized psychiatry. *International Journal of Eating Disorders, 45,* 70–78.

Striegel-Moore, R. H., Wilson, G. T., DeBar, L., Perrin, N., Lynch, F., Rosselli, F., et al. (2010). Cognitive behavioral guided self-help for the treatment of recurrent binge eating. *Journal of Consulting and Clinical Psychology, 78,* 312–321.

Wilson, G. T., & Zandberg, L. J. (2012). Cognitive-behavioral guided self-help for eating disorders: Effectiveness and scalability. *Clinical Psychology Review, 32,* 343–357.

Index

About the Author

Christopher G. Fairburn, DM, FMedSci, FRCPsych, is Wellcome Principal Research Fellow and Professor of Psychiatry at the University of Oxford. He directs the Centre for Research on Eating Disorders at Oxford (CREDO). Dr. Fairburn is a research clinician who has won many awards, including the Aaron T. Beck Award from the Academy of Cognitive Therapy and the Outstanding Researcher Award from the Academy for Eating Disorders. He has a particular interest in the global dissemination of effective psychological treatments. His website is *www.credo-oxford.com.*